The
Sexual Spectrum

Exploring
Human
Diversity

Olive Skene Johnson, Ph.D.

RAINCOAST BOOKS

Vancouver

Raincoast Books gratefully acknowledges the ongoing support of the Canada Council for the Arts, the British Columbia Arts Council and the Government of Canada through the Book Publishing Industry Development Program (BPIDP).

Cover design by Teresa Bubela
Interior design by Val Speidel

Library and Archives Canada Cataloguing in Publication

Johnson, Olive Skene, 1929-
        Sexual spectrum / Olive Skene Johnson.
Includes index.
ISBN 13: 978-1-55192-980-4
ISBN 10: 1-55192-980-5
        1. Sexual orientation. 2. Gender identity. 3. Sex differences. I. Title.

BF692.2.J64 2007   306.76   C2006-905242-5

Library of Congress Control Number: 2006937073

Raincoast Books
9050 Shaughnessy Street
Vancouver, British Columbia
Canada v6p 6e5
www.raincoast.com

In the United States:
Publishers Group West
1700 Fourth Street
Berkeley, California
94710

Raincoast Books is committed to protecting the environment and to the responsible use of natural resources. We are working with suppliers and printers to phase out our use of paper produced from ancient forests. This book is printed with vegetable-based inks on 100% ancient-forest-free, 100% post-consumer recycled, processed chlorine- and acid-free paper. For further information, visit our website at www.raincoast.com/publishing.

Printed in Canada by Webcom

10 9 8 7 6 5 4 3 2 1

PRAISE FOR THE SEXUAL SPECTRUM

"The book is so well-written the reader is unaware of being educated. Nevertheless, upon closing its covers, you have toured current research, scholarly opinion and political debate surrounding sexual diversity."

— *Globe and Mail*

"Lucid and methodical, this timely and reassuring book casts an eloquent light on a complex aspect of human experience that's still often relegated to dark corners; surprisingly so, given that we live in a sex-saturated society. Olive Skene Johnson takes a steady, even-handed approach to her examination of why sexuality is so gloriously polychromatic, and presents these variations as a logical, inevitable and morally neutral aspect of what it is to be human: man or woman, gay or straight, or standing contendedly on any of the many intermediary rungs."

— Bill Richardson

"*The Sexual Spectrum* is an ambitious attempt to explain the physiological, emotional and social bases for sexual differences in the world."

— *The Edmonton Journal*

"One of the best primers on gender, sex orientation and variations ever published."

— *LSB Review*

"Readers will come away with heightened appreciation for the kaleidoscopic variety of our species."

— *Quill & Quire*

"Olive Skene Johnson's *Sexual Spectrum* covers a range of topics and issues in the areas of sex, gender and sexuality, taking on everything from family dynamics, to neurobiology, to psychotherapy with equal vigour."

— *Herizons*

"Dr. Johnson's clear prose makes the latest findings in human sexuality accessible to everyone. Both objective and empathic, she carefully unravels the evidence for the biological and social sources of our sexual diversity, helping us to understand our own sexuality and that of other people. *The Sexual Spectrum* should be required reading!"

— Carolyn Harley, Ph.D., Professor of Psychology and Physiology, Memorial University

"This book is a highly readable and convenient introduction to a suite of inter-related topics including sex differences in the brain, sexual orientation, and gender identity. As a neuropsychologist, Olive Skene Johnson has one foot in the biological sciences and one in the social sciences, making her especially well suited to explain her subject. Johnson seamlessly weaves together her scientific knowledge and real-life experience into a coherent account of human sexual behaviour."

— Ray Blanchard, Ph.D., Head of Clinical Sexology Services, Centre for Addiction and Mental Health, and Professor of Psychiatry, Faculty of Medicine, University of Toronto *for Marc and Chris, who inspired this book*

The beauty of a quilt lies in the variety of its pieces.

ANON.

Contents

Introduction   1

1   MALENESS AND FEMALENESS   5
Feminine men and masculine women   11
Determinism — biological and social   12
Male and female hormones   14
Male and female brains   16
Four unusual human syndromes   16
Maleness and femaleness are separate qualities   20
BRAINSEX TEST   22
Sex is not just for reproduction   24
SEXUAL ORIENTATION QUIZ   28
Five facets of sexuality   30

2   SEXING THE BRAIN   33
Adam and Eve revisited   34
Brains are not sexually neutral   36
Structural and functional differences between male and
     female brains   38
Right brain/left brain — sex differences   43
Sex differences in cognitive abilities   47
Sex differences in communication and relationship   51
Sex differences in behaviour   52
The role of testosterone   54
Peculiar physical differences between the sexes   57
Sex differences in health outcomes   59
Sex differences in mate selection   61

3   MULTIPLE SEXUALITIES — THE MAJORS   63
Heterosexuals   64
Erotic attraction, not behaviour   65
So what do heterosexuals do?   66
Swingers   70
Transvestites   75
Paraphiliacs   76

Homosexuals   79
Homosexuality is worldwide   80
How many homosexuals are there?   81
Different types of homosexuality   89
Are gay men oversexed?   90
Drag queens and female impersonators   91
Do families "cause" homosexuality?   92
Gay and lesbian parents   95
What keeps homosexuality in the human gene pool?   103
Lesbians   105
Four sexes instead of two?   112

4   MULTIPLE SEXUALITIES — THE MINORS   113
Bisexuals   113
A bisexual woman's story   116
Are bisexuals more highly sexed?   119
Bisexual men versus women   119
Bisexual politics   121

Transsexuals   122
How Catherine became David   125
Making a woman out of a man, and vice versa   130
Treatment outcomes   135

Intersexuals   140
How Danny became Danielle   143
The "John/Joan" case   147
Sexual identity is inborn   149
Changing doctors' attitudes   151

5   DIFFERENT BRAINS FOR DIFFERENT SEXUALITIES   153
Gay brains and straight brains   155
Behavioural differences between gays and straights   159
Differences in cognitive abilities   162
Other differences between gays and straights   164
Transsexual brains   169
What about brain differences *within* groups?   171

6   BIOLOGY AND SEXUAL ORIENTATION   172
Is biology destiny?   172
The gene theory of sexual orientation   174
Homosexuality in families   177
The maternal immune hypothesis   181
The neuroendocrine theory of sexual orientation   183
Does prenatal stress affect sexual orientation?   184
Developmental instability   186
Bias, not predestination   187

7   NATURE AND NURTURE — THE DANCE GOES ON   189
Is sexual orientation "constructed"?   190
The interactionist view   192
Interactions among genes, hormones and environment   201
Which environment?   202
Two indirect models of sexual orientation   205
The dance goes on   208

8   IF IT'S NORMAL, WHY ALL THE FUSS?   *210*
Intolerance — private and public   210
Are gay-bashers secretly gay?   214
The myth that "majority means normal"   215
The myth that homosexuals are sick and the myth that
    homosexuality is just a preference   215
Stereotypes   216
"Curing" homosexuality   218
Religious opposition   221
The winds of change   226
Legal rights for sexual minorities in the U.S.   228
Legal rights for sexual minorities in Canada   236
Legal rights for sexual minorities elsewhere   242
Familiarity breeds tolerance   245

Acknowledgements   249
Bibliography   251
Permissions   269
Index   272
About the author   277

Introduction

SOME YEARS AGO, when I was attending a workshop on sexuality, I was asked to imagine myself in love with a woman. Gay men and lesbians in the workshop were asked to imagine themselves in love with someone of the opposite sex. I closed my eyes and an image of my friend F popped into my mind. She and I have known each other for years, shared the trials and triumphs of parenting, fought election campaigns together, grieved for her dead husband and my dead son, immersed ourselves in wonderful summer courses at Oxford and Cambridge. If I were to fall in love with any woman, I imagine it would be F, whom I already love anyway.

Yet, try as I might to imagine being *in* love with her, I could not. I could get as far as imagining the two of us setting up house and doing all the homey things couples do — reading, watching TV, decorating the house, going to concerts, talking about our kids, cooking together. But to be sexually involved with F? Impossible. Ridiculous. Though I knew F loved me as a friend, I also knew she would fall down in hysterical laughter at the very mention of our being lovers.

Abandoning the notion of F as lover, I tried to conjure up a stranger to mentally fall in love with, but that proved impossible, too. How could I fall in love with some woman I didn't even know or care about, and who didn't know me?

When the workshop exercise ended, I discovered that most straight-people had encountered the same problems I did. The gay men and lesbians in the group were somewhat more successful, since most of them had had some heterosexual experience when they were younger, before they declared themselves as gay. Even so, they still found the exercise difficult.

Then the workshop leader asked us to imagine falling in love with someone who was the same sex as our mates or partners. This time when I closed my eyes I immediately thought of my favourite movie star, Paul Newman (remember, this was some time ago). With no effort at all, I imagined myself swooning in his arms, gazing into those amazing blue eyes, thrilling to his kisses.

But hold it, Paul doesn't know me any better than that strange woman I imagined a minute ago does. And apart from his movies, I don't know him, either. So why is it so easy for me to imagine being in love with Paul even though I'm already in love with my husband? Could it be precisely *because* I'm already in love with a man?

When the exercise ended, I learned that my experience was pretty typical of the group. Almost everybody had found it easy to imagine being in love with someone of the sex they normally loved, whereas they'd found it difficult or impossible to feel in love with the other sex. People described the latter as feeling "unnatural," "not me," even "distasteful."

What is it that distinguishes the kind of love we feel for cherished friends from the kind we feel when we're in love? The most obvious difference, of course, is that being in love involves sexual attraction, which doesn't enter the picture in platonic love. Friend-love is about shared experience, mutual understanding and liking, and lending emotional support. What it's not about is sex. People in love can also be best friends, of course. On the other hand, being sexually attracted to someone doesn't guarantee that you're in love. But *unless* you're sexually attracted, you can't be in love with the nicest person in the world.

What is it that makes most people feel sexual toward one sex but not the other? Why is a minority of people sexually attracted only to its own sex? And what about people who love both sexes? Why are there differences in how masculine or feminine people are? Why are some women very masculine and some men very feminine? Can a woman really change into a man?

Why do some men like to dress in women's clothing? What happens when a baby is born with genitals of both sexes? Do children raised by homosexuals become gay? Why do gay men tend to have more older brothers than straight men? Are there really more than two sexes?

The answers involve a radical new understanding of sexuality, one that goes beyond simple either–ors like male–female and gay–straight. The new model reflects the fact that each of us is a unique combination of genes, sex hormones, genitals, inner identity, erotic orientation and psychological masculinity and femininity. Together we comprise a vast array of sex and gender differences, some obvious and some subtle, that make up the human family. That diversity is the story of this book.

A *note on terminology*: For convenience, I sometimes use the colloquial terms "gay" for homosexual and "straight" for heterosexual. When I use the term "gender," it's to refer only to a person's social role — that is, which of the set of social and cultural characteristics considered appropriate either for men or for women does this person display? This was always the meaning of "gender" in the past, while "sex" was used to indicate the person's male or female body and inner identity. Today, however, "gender" is confusingly applied to a variety of things, including physical sex and sexual identity. The word has also acquired political meanings. For the sake of clarity, therefore, "sex" is used here to denote the physical body and the person's identity as male or female, while "gender" denotes the person's social role.

In discussing people whose physical bodies are at odds with their sexual identities, I use the word "transsexual" rather than "transgender," again for clarity. "Transgender" is often used nowadays to refer to people who live as the other sex but have not had sex-change surgery. However, many of these people have had hormonal treatments if not surgery, or else breast surgery but not surgical removal of the penis, and so their transition, while incomplete, involves more than simply dressing and living as the other sex. To avoid confusion, therefore, I use the term "transsexual" for all people whose sexual identity is at variance with their bodies, whether or not they have had sex-change surgery.

When describing differences between men and women, and between straight and gay people, I am always referring to *average* differences, which of course don't reveal anything about any particular person. For every sex difference described, there will be some women who score higher than some men, and vice versa. The same is true for differences between gays and straights. Some gay people will obtain scores more like those of straight people, while some straights will obtain scores more like those of gays. That's why you can't jump to conclusions about yourself or your mate on the basis of reported averages.

The interviews in this book were conducted before the book was written but are presented in the present tense for dramatic impact. Some of the personal information reported in these interviews may have changed.

Papers, books and studies referred to in each chapter are listed in the bibliography at the back of the book.

1

Maleness and Femaleness

Men are born equal but they are also born different.

ERICH FROMM, *Escape from Freedom*

M Y FAMILY is a collection of minorities. My youngest son, who's adopted, is of mixed race and looks black. One daughter is left-handed, making her part of a 10 percent minority. Two older sons are gay, members of an even smaller minority.

Thankfully, our adopted son has suffered very little racial discrimination. When it did occur, it was usually from the police: as a teenager returning home in the evening, Mike was several times stopped for questioning. Their excuse was always the same: "A robbery has been reported, and the suspect answers your description." We used to laugh (after our anger had cooled) because at that time there was nobody else answering Mike's description in our entire white middle-class neighbourhood.

Apart from the police, there were only minor incidents, such as the time when Mike was 16 and we were going through a Cairo museum and suddenly realized he had disappeared. After a frantic search, we discovered him being hauled outside by two museum guards who had mistaken him for an Arab gate-crasher (he was wearing a checkered Arab head scarf he'd just bought in a bazaar). Other times, going through airline boarding procedures, Mike always received tougher scrutiny than the rest of us. But apart from such isolated incidents, his race has never been much of an issue.

Same thing for our daughter's unusual hand usage. We've often said how thankful we are that she was born in the late 20th century and not a few centuries earlier, when left-handers were believed to be cursed — bad luck at best and witches at worst. It's no coincidence that the word "sinistral" (meaning "left") is from the Latin "sinister," meaning evil. Many of these unfortunate sinistrals ended up being tortured or burned at the stake. Mercifully, by the time the 20th century arrived, society had stopped killing left-handers, but even then well-meaning parents and teachers were still trying to "cure" them (just as today some well-meaning therapists still try to "cure" homosexuals). They would tie the child's left hand behind her back, forcing her to use the other hand. Not only did these children's handwriting suffer, but some of them became stutterers as well. (It was not known then that in most people the brain is "wired" a certain way to control both the writing hand and spoken language, and disrupting these arrangements can sometimes cause stuttering.)

Worst of all, left-handers became imbued at an early age with a sense of shame. Not about anything they'd done, but about what they *were*. If their parents failed to make this clear, then their teachers often would. When the child arrived at school, he learned that being left-handed was unacceptable, unnatural, bad. Something that had to be "cured." As adults, left-handers might laugh off the humiliation they had endured, perhaps apologizing for their poor handwriting. But early shaming can have long-lasting effects despite later attempts to make light of it, so we're grateful that our daughter didn't have to go through that.

Our gay sons were not so fortunate. Prejudice against racial and other minorities was steadily decreasing when they were growing up, but prejudice against sexual minorities was still the norm. Gay teachers remained well closeted (anything else would have cost them their jobs); homosexuals had almost zero public visibility. Though sexual activity between two men or two women in Canada was decriminalized in 1969, it was still perfectly legal to discriminate against them in immigration, employment, military service, housing, pensions and other benefits, marriage and custody of children. Stories of gay-bashing appeared frequently in the daily newspaper and the perpetrators were almost never caught, let alone charged. Being gay in North America (and most other places) was a very risky circumstance.

I still remember the day we learned that our eldest son, Marcus, was gay. He was 22 years old and had just moved into an apartment with another young man whom we'd not yet met. His father and I were invited to dinner to meet Marc's roommate. When they announced during pre-dinner drinks that they were "an item," my initial shock was followed by a whirlwind of confused thoughts. "My God, this means that people will start treating Marc like a leper — he could even be beaten or killed!" I felt as though my heart would thump right out of my chest. Breathing deeply to calm myself down, I managed to get my terror under control, but that was quickly replaced by feelings of profound sadness: this must mean that Marc would never have children. I felt deeply, despairingly sorry for him. How on earth could this have happened?

But the look on Marc's face was not in the least sad. In fact, he looked happy, even joyous. He actually appeared delighted to be making this important announcement to us. It was obvious that a heavy burden had been lifted from him. He was in love and he wanted to share his good news with us. He trusted us to receive the news as kindred spirits. Somehow we managed a smile and a hug, but the rest of the evening went by in a kind of blur. I do remember thinking during the dinner, "This will probably pass (as many of Marc's other crazy adventures had) but meanwhile it's pretty interesting." I was fascinated by the roommate, a handsome, articulate man whose manner was quite effeminate. I realized I had never actually known a gay man "up close and personal."

I can honestly say that neither my husband nor I ever saw our son's gayness as a moral issue, not on that day nor ever after. We had drilled into our children our belief that everyone is important and everyone's differences deserve respect. Bigotry was an evil force to be resisted wherever it raised its ugly head. We had never felt ill will toward homosexual people; we had felt sad for them, believing that their lives must be very difficult and wondering why they had turned out like that.

And so our feelings were more of the "where did we go wrong?" variety.

It simply never occurred to us that perhaps this had nothing to do with us. After all, we were his parents; we had been the biggest influence on his life, so it must be our fault.

More accurately, it must be *my* fault. I was clearly the one to point the finger at, in an era when child-rearing was a mother's full-time job. Maybe I had been too busy with outside activities? I should have been paying more attention to what was happening at home.

Shortly afterward I read a book called *Mother, I Have Something to Tell You*, by Jo Brans, which describes the feelings of parents whose children, after the 1960s, did not turn out as expected. A quotation in the book (from Alison Lurie's novel *The War between the Tates*) sprang out at me. Erica Tate, whose children (with the unlikely names of Muffy and Jeffo) are "going from bad to worse," is thinking the same way I was thinking after Marc announced that he was gay.

The worst part of it all is that the children are her fault. All the authorities and writers say so. In their innocent past Erica and

Brian had blamed their own shortcomings on their parents while retaining credit for their own achievements. They had passed judgement on the character of acquaintances whose young children were not as nice as Muffy and Jeffo — but everyone did that. To have had disagreeable parents excused one's faults; to have disagreeable children underlined them. The parents might not look especially guilty; they might seem outwardly to be intelligent, kind and charming people — but inside were Mr. and Mrs. Hyde.

It was agreed everywhere, also, that Mrs. Hyde was the worse, or at least the more responsible ... After all ... [the children] were in her "area of operations."

Our eldest son grew up during the turbulent sixties and the hip seventies, when young people were bombarded with music and messages urging them to "let it all hang out," "do your own thing," "don't trust anybody over thirty." Marc eagerly heeded the messages. He demonstrated against the Vietnam war, grew long hair, experimented with drugs, dropped out of university, dreamed of Utopia. For traditional parents, the era was a nightmare. Even for liberal parents it was a tough time, never knowing whether we were being too liberal or not liberal enough, terrified that our bright, promising kids were ruining their lives. We reminded ourselves that each generation has the right to evolve its own set of values, but in the small hours of the night, lying awake staring at the ceiling, we were scared.

In light of the rebellious tenor of the times, we initially interpreted Marc's "coming out" as just one more rebellious act. It didn't help when he insisted that being gay was a political statement and a personal choice (he later changed his mind about this). If he could choose to be gay, why couldn't he just choose to be straight again? His failure to do so seemed to us like more adolescent acting out. For a while I secretly entertained the hope that eventually he would come to his senses, quit being gay and marry some nice young woman who would have babies — our grandchildren!

Yes, I have to confess that, after the first surprise of Marc's announcement wore off, I started feeling as sorry for my husband and myself as I did for Marc. Poor Marc, never to know the joys of fatherhood, and poor us, robbed of the joy of seeing his genes (and ours) living on in our grandchildren. I comforted myself with the knowledge that our other children would surely give us grandchildren, but that didn't make up for Marc's loss. Why was he being so foolish?

By the time our second son announced that he was gay, some years later, we were a lot smarter. I had gone back to graduate school and earned a Ph.D. in psychology. I learned that sex hormones can sometimes make animals act like the opposite sex. I read about human syndromes that appeared to do the same thing. I learned that men's and women's brains are not the same. I wondered whether that might also be true of gays and straights. I wanted to know more.

Since then, I have read everything I could get my hands on about homosexuality and about other sexual orientations and identities. And I realize now how naïve most of us have been. We have been reluctant even to recognize the important differences between men and women, let alone the numerous shades of maleness and femaleness, and of erotic attractions, that are subsumed by "male" and "female."

I have learned that we have to move past simple either/ors like male/female and gay/straight. As scientists discover more and more about human development and human behaviour, it's becoming increasingly obvious that human sexuality is much closer to a complex mosaic than it is to simple either/ors. There are too many things that can't be explained by those catch-all categories.

"Male/female" cannot explain why, in widely differing cultures around the world, there are always men who are attracted to men and women who are attracted to women. Nor can it explain why some seemingly ordinary men sometimes like to dress up in women's clothing, or why in all cultures some men and some women are attracted to both males *and* females, and some women and men inwardly identify as the opposite sex. "Gay/straight" cannot explain why some heterosexual men are effeminate and some heterosexual women are very masculine. Nor can it explain why there are various kinds of gay or straight people, some masculine, some feminine, others a mixture of both. And none of these labels — male/female/gay/straight — can accurately describe cross-dressers or transsexuals or people born with ambiguous genitals or other physical anomalies that defy the usual sexual categorizations. Obviously we need a new way of looking at differences in human sexuality.

FEMININE MEN AND MASCULINE WOMEN

All of us have at some time or other known at least one man who was married, had fathered children, held an okay job and was in all respects perfectly unexceptional except that he seemed even more feminine than most of our female friends. I had a friend like that. He was a high school teacher who designed his wife's clothes and made her hats; he loved to cook and try out new recipes (at a time when most men didn't cook); he happily shared in the child care (at a time when men rarely changed diapers). "But wasn't he really gay?" you may wonder. No, he was not. I know that, because we were close enough as friends to talk about everything. He loved his wife deeply and passionately, and had no sexual longing for anyone else, male or female. Neither did he appear to have any significant psychological problems. He was certainly different from most of the men I knew, but he was a happy man, content with his family and his life generally.

Haven't you also known at least one woman whose interests and behaviour were exactly the opposite of my hat-making friend? Mine was a woman who almost always wore overalls (in the days when only farm women did). After she had children and became a stay-at-home mom, she built new kitchen cupboards and enjoyed doing plumbing and other repairs around the house. She handled the family's finances and made most of the important family decisions.

She was highly intellectual and had no interest whatsoever in talking about feelings or exchanging gossip. She was married to a rather effeminate man who shared her intellectual interests. In their differences they appeared to complement one another and their marriage appeared to be very successful.

So what should we think about individuals such as these, who are practising heterosexuals but who do not fit the usual pattern of heterosexual male or female behaviour? How did they get that way anyway? Did their parents raise them in unusual ways? If so, why did my effeminate friend's brother, 18 months younger than he, turn out to be just a typical kind of guy? And why didn't my masculine female friend turn out to be more like the sisters she was raised with?

Are mannish women and effeminate men unnatural oddballs, distinctly different from the rest of us, or are they in fact just two of the many possible normal variations on the male/female theme? If the latter, how does such variety in human beings occur?

DETERMINISM — BIOLOGICAL AND SOCIAL

Two diametrically opposed theories of human behaviour have been waging war for several decades. The biological determinists argue that human behaviour, including sexual behaviour, flows directly from our biology, mainly from the effects of our genes. The opposing opinion — that of the social constructionists — claims that people's behaviour is "constructed" from their family environment, the culture they live in, the friends they have, and the myriad other social influences to which they are exposed.

I reject both of these positions. In my view the biological determinists err in attributing a *causal* role to genes, rather than an *enabling* role. Genes code for specific proteins, not for behaviours or psychological characteristics. Except for single genes that are involved in traits such as hair and eye colour, or in certain diseases such as cystic fibrosis and Huntington's disease, genes exert *indirect*, not direct, effects. And complex human traits like sexual identity and sexual orientation probably require the interaction of many genes, in complex ways not yet well understood.

But though genes don't *cause* behaviour, they do play an important role in it. Without genes, nothing is possible. Making possible, in fact, is what genes do. They allow for things to happen; they set the stage for behaviour but they don't always force the actors onto the stage. Sometimes genes make it highly *likely* that a behaviour will occur, but they don't guarantee it.

Social constructionists, in my view, err in the same black-and-white way as the biological determinists, except that they attribute a causal role to social factors instead of genetic ones. They argue that there's nothing biologically innate about sexual identity and sexual orientation; it's social experience alone that produces sex differences and different sexual orientations. These people are social determinists just as their opposites are biological determinists.

I don't accept either of these views. I believe there is convincing evidence (which I'll share with you in future chapters) that human personality and behaviour, including sexual behaviour, develop from an *interaction* between biological and social factors: it's not biology or society that calls the shots, it's both. Without biological predisposition, it's unlikely that you would ever be able to develop certain characteristics, including sexual traits. On the other hand, whether or not your inherent predisposition for a certain trait will ever get expressed in your behaviour depends on your social experiences, probably to a greater or lesser degree in different individuals. You may be a person who is extremely vulnerable to the effects of social influences, whereas your best friend may be quite the opposite. Also, certain traits have been shown to be more amenable to social influence, while other traits stubbornly resist it.

Later chapters will discuss both the biological and the social evidence for sexual identity and sexual orientation. But first, a look at how we get to be sexual beings in the first place, and why there is such a range of femaleness and maleness.

MALE AND FEMALE HORMONES

We hear a lot these days about the "male" hormone, testosterone, and the "female" hormones, estrogen and progesterone. In fact, both males and females have all three of these hormones. All of them start out as cholesterol and then, in a series of biochemical steps, enzymes in the testes and ovaries change the cholesterol into the various sex hormones.

Though all three of these hormones occur in both men and women, each sex has a different ratio of them. Women produce more estrogen and progesterone than men but their ovaries and adrenal glands also produce smaller amounts of testosterone. Men produce more testosterone than females but they also produce smaller amounts of estrogen and progesterone.

As a fetus develops in the womb, circulating sex hormones act upon the neural circuits of its brain, creating a permanently male or female brain. Typically the sex of an infant's brain is in line with the genetic sex dictated by its chromosomes, but this is not always the case, as we'll see in later chapters. And even when body sex and brain sex are consistent with one another, as they usually are, there can still be various *shades* of maleness and femaleness laid down in the fetal brain. That's because exposure to hormones in the womb is not an either/or event; its effect depends on several factors: *How much* hormone exposure was there? *How long* did it last? What was the *ratio* of male-to-female sex hormones? *Exactly when* did the hormone exposure take place?

In addition, what peculiarities does this fetus have that will help determine its brain's unique response to the various sex hormones? Are there too few receptors (on the surface of its neurons) for a particular hormone? Are the receptors low in sensitivity for that hormone? If so, the fetus' brain will be unable to make use of that hormone, no matter how much of it is circulating. Even when there are enough receptors and their sensitivity is high, any fetus' *response* to that hormone will depend on its individual genetic makeup. Two fetuses may receive exactly the same hormones, in the same amounts, and at the same times, yet each will be affected differently.

For all these reasons, every developing brain receives unique doses of each of the sex hormones. It's obvious then, that a variety of outcomes should result. Different outcomes can occur from larger or smaller doses of hormone, from different combinations of hormones, from brief or lengthy exposure to a hormone, or from receiving a hormone at different points during gestation. Various outcomes can also result from genetic differences in each fetus, and differences in the number and sensitivity of the receptors on its neurons.

Every one of us, during our earliest development, receives a unique exposure to the sex hormones that sculpt the neural circuits in our brains. This implies that *every person's brain — and by inference everyone's later behaviour — starts out as some unique combination of male and female, masculine and feminine.*

Do these early hormones affect our erotic orientation as well as our inner sexuality? According to the neuroendocrine theory of sexuality (see Chapter 6), they do. This theory claims that at puberty, sex hormones once again flowing through the system activate the effects of what was previously organized in the brain during gestation or shortly afterward.

Psychologist/sexologist John Money, author of *Gay, Straight, and In-Between,* explains it this way: "The hormones of puberty mature the body and activate in the mind the erotic sensualism that is already programmed therein ... Pubertal adolescents do not choose their erotic sensualism. They encounter it, as preformed in the mind." Sounds as though Money is saying that people's sexual orientation is permanently set by their early hormones. In fact, Money is careful to talk about a *proclivity* for sexual orientation, not a predestination: "Many wrongly assume that whatever is biological cannot be changed, and whatever mental can be. Both propositions are in error." But that's a topic for later chapters. First, more about how early sex hormones acting on our brains can affect our later adult behaviour.

MALE AND FEMALE BRAINS

Some of the earliest clues about brain sex came from experiments involving laboratory animals. Of course there are important differences between humans and animals, so we can't automatically apply the findings from animal studies to humans. But animal studies are still very valuable because in many respects human brains closely resemble the brains of certain animals. The results of animal studies often provide tantalizing leads to be followed up with studies of humans.

In animals the brain's sex is inferred from the animal's behaviour, chiefly its mating behaviour. Male animals typically mount females, and female animals typically present themselves for sex in a posture known as lordosis, in which the back is bent and the rump is elevated. In a wide variety of experiments in various animal species, when scientists have changed the levels of early sex hormones, the animals' mating behaviours have been altered to be more like those of the opposite sex. Male animals can be induced to display lordosis, and female animals can be induced to mount, if their sex hormones are altered at critical periods before birth or shortly afterward. Regardless of an animal's genetic sex, its brain can be permanently altered by sex hormones given at critical early periods, and this will make the animal in adulthood behave as though it were a member of the opposite sex.

What about humans? Human brains, of course, can't be doused with male or female hormones so that scientists can learn how this treatment affects the person's later behaviour. But several naturally occurring human syndromes do provide us with evidence of the effect of prenatal hormones on people.

FOUR UNUSUAL HUMAN SYNDROMES

In an inherited condition known as CAH (congenital adrenal hyperplasia), female infants are born with an enzyme deficiency that causes their adrenal glands to produce excessive amounts of male hormones before birth and shortly afterward. The effect of this is similar to the effect on experimental animals who've received excess testosterone during early development — that is, their later behaviour was less feminine and more masculine than it typically would have been. In childhood most CAH females are more tomboyish — more physical, more active, more daring — than other girls. They prefer boys' toys, games and hobbies over the activities usually preferred by girls. They're more interested in competitive sports. On tests of spatial ability, they score as high as boys do, and much higher than other girls.

In adulthood, CAH women often have a more masculine appearance than other women. They tend to be more aggressive and, most interesting of all, there's an increased incidence of homosexual and bisexual orientation among them. They also have an increased likelihood of being left-handed and of having very good spatial abilities, both of which occur in men more often than in women. As well, CAH women have a masculine finger-length pattern — index finger shorter than ring finger — whereas in most women the two fingers are about the same length (more about that later).

In another condition known as AIS (androgen insensitivity syndrome), male fetuses have malfunctioning receptors for androgen (male sex hormone) and therefore they can't make use of the androgen that's produced by their testes and circulating in their bodies. In consequence, their bodies and brains don't get masculinized. They are born with female genitals, look like girl babies and are reared as girls. These AIS "girls" are often not diagnosed until they fail to menstruate and are taken to a doctor to see why. An examination reveals that they have no uterus, no Fallopian tubes and no ovaries.

As adults, AIS women identify as female and their erotic orientation is toward men. But these are generally not ordinary women; instead, they tend to be hyperfeminine, wanting only to get married and stay home looking after husbands and children, rather than going out to work or making their mark in the world some other way. Lacking the small amounts of male hormones that other women

have to balance their plentiful estrogen, many AIS women go over-
board on femininity.

A third group of infants who received abnormal amounts of prenatal hormones were those girls whose pregnant mothers received
DES (diethylstilbestrol), the first synthetic estrogen ever made. DES
was widely used between 1947 and 1971 to prevent miscarriage in at-
risk pregnancies. By the time it was banned in 1971, hundreds of
thousands of pregnant women had been prescribed the hormone by
their physicians. It's now known that DES affects fetal brain tissues,
making them more masculine and less feminine. When girls who'd
been exposed to DES in the womb grew up, they had more male-
typical behaviours and fewer female-typical behaviours, compared to
women who had not been exposed. DES women still identified as
female, but like the CAH women, there was an increased incidence
of homosexual and bisexual orientation among them. They also had
a higher incidence of left-handedness (as men have), especially if
their exposure to DES occurred early in gestation. If exposure
occurred late in gestation, they were more likely to have a male pattern in the way their brains processed verbal information. (These
kinds of male/female differences are discussed in the next chapter.)

In addition to these brain effects, DES-exposed daughters (now in
their 30s, 40s and 50s) have suffered physical effects. They're more
susceptible to certain cancers and to malformations of the reproductive organs. They also have increased rates of infertility, ectopic pregnancy, miscarriage and premature labour.

In the sons of DES mothers, the effect of DES was feminizing:
despite having a typical male upbringing, these boys had extremely
feminine behaviours. In adulthood they've experienced a number of
problems. These include low sperm counts and genital malformations, including underdeveloped or undescended testicles. An
increased risk of prostate cancer is also suspected. Even more alarm-
ing, animal experiments have now shown that the harmful effects of
DES may continue into the third generation (the grandchildren of

the original DES mothers), who may be at increased risk of developing reproductive-tract tumours and other rare tumours.

The fourth syndrome involving abnormal amounts of sex hormone in the womb is an inherited disorder, 5-alpha Reductase Deficiency, a profound enzyme deficiency that interferes with fetal testosterone. Boy babies are born with female-like genitals and are usually raised as girls. This disorder was quite common, due to inbreeding, in a remote rural area of the Dominican Republic where scientists studied these children. At puberty, when their bodies produced testosterone, these "girls" became masculinized: their voice deepened, their shoulders broadened, and their penises developed. All but one of them then abandoned the female role and name; they married women and assumed men's work. Outside of the Dominican Republic, where the disorder is quite rare, affected individuals usually have their testicles removed before puberty so they are not exposed to the surge of pubertal testosterone that would masculinize them. This enables them to live as females throughout their lives.

All of the conditions described above show what can happen when people have been exposed to abnormal amounts of sex hormones in the womb. These syndromes are unusual, and so the number of people affected by them is very small. Unfortunately, the same can't be said for the number of infants affected by various commonly abused drugs ingested by their parents. Alcohol, nicotine, marijuana, heroin, cocaine, amphetamines and other drugs taken during pregnancy can all affect early fetal development. Studies show that males generally are more severely affected than females. Among other things, drugs can suppress the level of testosterone in a male fetus, causing reduced masculinization — that is, having fewer male physical and mental characteristics. Drugs can also cause incomplete defeminization in a male fetus — that is, it retains some female characteristics both physically and mentally. (As the section below explains, making a fetus masculine is not the same thing as making it less feminine.)

MALENESS AND FEMALENESS ARE SEPARATE QUALITIES

Until the early 1970s, it was believed that maleness and femaleness were arranged on a continuum: the more you had of one, the less you'd have of the other. This belief was based on studies in which researchers altered an animal's hormone levels at sensitive periods in its development and then observed any changes in its mating behaviour when it reached adulthood. For example, when researchers gave testosterone to pregnant guinea pigs, the female offspring of these guinea pigs had abnormal adult sexual behaviour. Instead of displaying lordosis like normal females, they behaved like mating males. Experimenters concluded that giving testosterone to pregnant animals had pushed the offspring over to the male end of the sexual spectrum.

Subsequently, however, it became clear that maleness and femaleness were not opposite ends of a spectrum, but were actually independent of one another. Scientists learned that treating animals with hormones during development could defeminize their behaviour *without* masculinizing it — that is, females would stop doing their normal female things, but that didn't mean they would start doing male-type things. The opposite was also true. Female animals could be induced to start doing male-type things without losing their ability to do their regular female-type things. For example, when pregnant ewes were implanted with testosterone at different points in gestation, some of their offspring mounted like males while *also* displaying lordosis like females. This meant that their brains were *both* masculine and feminine. Other offspring showed *only* male behaviour or *only* female behaviour. Which of these outcomes would happen depended on just when during gestation the pregnant ewe received the testosterone.

In later experiments, researchers made an amazing discovery: the brain actually has two separate neural pathways for masculine and feminine behaviour. Working with newborn rats, researchers implanted tiny pellets of estradiol (a kind of estrogen) into the hypothalamus, a tiny structure at the base of the brain that is known to be involved in male and female mating behaviour. When the hormone was implanted on the left side of the newborn's hypothalamus, it defeminized the animal's brain, which had the effect of suppressing female mating behaviour when the animal grew to adulthood. When the hormone was implanted on the right side of the newborn's hypothalamus, it masculinized the animal's brain, which increased male mating behaviour in adulthood. What's surprising about these two neural systems is that they appear to operate independently: activating one does not automatically shut down the other. That's what happened with some of the female offspring of the hormonally treated ewes. Their brains were masculinized (which induced them to mount other females) without being defeminized (as shown by the fact that they still assumed the female lordosis posture).

What about humans? Is one part of our brain masculine and another part femine? And how about homosexual men? Are their brains masculinized without being defeminized?

Nobody can definitively answer these questions yet, but interestingly, psychologists have found that people's masculine and feminine psychological characteristics are independent of one another. On checklists measuring a person's degree of psychological masculinity and femininity, the person gets two scores, one for the degree of masculinity and one for the degree of femininity. You can be high on one and low on the other if you're either very masculine or very feminine, or you can be high on both if you're a highly androgynous person, low on both if you're asexual, or somewhere in the middle of both.

The trouble with psychological checklists is that cultural norms for masculine and feminine behaviour change over time. Some of what was considered appropriately feminine and masculine for Western women and men in the 1950s would be laughed at today in the light of greater equality between the sexes. And so, to get away from measuring stereotypical male and female personality characteristics,

British geneticist Anne Moir designed a different kind of test. Instead of listing personality characteristics, this test is based on the different ways of thinking that have been identified between men and women (reviewed in the next chapter). These are believed to be related to differences in male and female brains. To see how typically male or female your own thinking is, take the test below.

❖ ————————————————————————— ❖

BRAINSEX TEST

(from *Brainsex*, by Anne Moir and David Jessel)

You hear an indistinct meow. Without looking around, how well can you place the cat?
- (a)   If you think about it, you can point to it.
- (b)   You can point straight to it.
- (c)   You don't know if you could point to it.

How good are you at remembering a song you've just heard?
- (a)   You find it easy and you can sing part of it in tune.
- (b)   You can only do it if it's simple and rhythmical.
- (c)   You find it difficult.

A person you've met a few times telephones you. How easy is it for you to recognize that voice in the few seconds before the person tells you who they are?
- (a)   You'd find it quite easy.
- (b)   You'd recognize the voice at least half the time.
- (c)   You'd recognize the voice less than half the time.

You're with a group of married friends. Two of them are having a clandestine affair. Would you detect their relationship?
- (a)   Nearly always

(b) Half the time

(c) Seldom

You're at a large and purely social gathering. You're introduced to five strangers. If their names are mentioned the following day, how easy is it for you to picture their faces?

(a) You'll remember most of them.

(b) You'll remember a few of them.

(c) You'll seldom remember any of them.

In your early school days how easy was spelling and the writing of essays?

(a) Both were quite easy.

(b) One was easy.

(c) Neither was easy.

You spot a parking place but you must reverse into it — and it's going to be a fairly tight squeeze:

(a) You look for another space.

(b) You back into it ... carefully.

(c) You reverse into it without much thought.

You've spent three days in a strange village and someone asks you which way is north:

(a) You're unlikely to know.

(b) You're not sure, but given a moment you can work it out.

(c) You point north.

You're in a dentist's waiting room with half a dozen people of the same sex as yourself. How close can you sit to one of them without feeling uncomfortable?

(a) less than 6 inches (15 cm)

(b) 6 inches to 2 feet (15 cm to 60 cm)

(c) more than 2 feet (60 cm plus)

You're visiting your new neighbour and the two of you are talking. There's a tap dripping gently in the background. Otherwise the room is quiet:

* (a)   You'd notice the dripping sound immediately and try to ignore it.
  (b)   If you noticed it, you'd probably mention it.
─ (c)   It doesn't bother you at all.

Scoring the test

Unanswered questions count for 5 points.

MALES   score 10 points for each (a)
             5 points for each (b)
             −5 points for each (c)
FEMALES   score 15 points for each (a)
             5 points for each (b)
             −5 points for each (c)

Most males will score between 0 and 60. Most females will score between 50 and 100. The overlap (scores between 50 and 60) indicates a thought compatibility between sexes.

Male scores below 0 and female scores above 100 point to a very differently "wired" brain from that of the opposite sex.

Male scores above 60 may show a brain sex bias to the female.

Females who score below 50 may show a brain sex bias to the male.

However, all such differences are average differences. A male might score above 60 and still possess a male brain. A female might score below 50 and still possess a female brain.

❖ ──────────────────────────────── ❖

SEX IS NOT JUST FOR REPRODUCTION

Part of what prevents us from recognizing a *variety* of sexualities is our historical habit of equating sex with reproduction. Jonathan Katz (*The Invention of Heterosexuality*) reports how, as late as the 1890s, the "sexual instinct" in people was still defined as "procreative desire." By the turn of the century, however, "sexual instinct" began to be recognized as erotic desire rather than as desire to procreate. Katz argues that the fall of the old reproductive ethic and the widespread use of birth control have eliminated the difference between hetero-sexuality and homosexuality: "The commodification of pleasure ... breaks down old distinctions between hetero and homo ... Few people now, except the Pope, judge the quality of heterosexual relations by their fecundity." (For more about breaking down distinctions between hetero and homo, see Swingers, Chapter 3, and Bisexuals, Chapter 4.)

Even in modern times the biomedical sciences have tended to downplay the erotic aspects of sex. Subjects such as infertility, gesta-tion and childbirth have been intensively studied while subjects such as eroticism, sexual lust and sexual orientation have been grossly neglected.

This tendency has affected animal scientists as well as human ones. Bruce Bagemihl (*Biological Exuberance*), himself a biologist, claims that same-sex behaviour in animals has been observed for many years but scientists, no matter how well-intentioned, looked at animals through culturally biased lenses: animals copulated in order to reproduce themselves. When these biologists observed animals engaging in non-reproductive sexual activity, says Bagemihl, they either ignored the behaviour and failed to report it in their profes-sional journals or else they reported it as one of Mother Nature's little mistakes. Often they renamed it as "aggression" or "appeasement" or some kind of "bonding" ritual, instead of sexual activity.

For example, Bagemihl notes, it has been known for many years that six to ten percent of male rams are homosexual — that is, they prefer to mount other male rams even when estrous females are present and available to them. Scientists noting the homosexual behaviour of these rams dismissed it as aggression. Despite the evi-dence of their own eyes, they were blinded by their firm belief that reproductive urge alone is what drives animals to sexual interactions. (Recent study of homosexual rams discovered that they actually have different hormone profiles from other rams and different hormone activities in certain parts of their brains, and these anomalies could explain their homosexual orientation.)

Fortunately, in recent years some animal biologists have begun to criticize the rigid sex-for-babies model. (It occurs to me that, if they'd been studying humans instead of animals, they might have recognized sooner what everybody else already knew — that most sexual activity has nothing to do with making babies!) Psychologist Paul Vasey of the University of Lethbridge reported that, in some populations of Japanese macaques, females routinely engage in both heterosexual and homosexual sex, and should properly be called bisexual. Females will choose specific same-sex partners over certain male mates, and vice versa. The researchers determined that the females' same-sex behaviour is truly sexual, rather than merely social.

Bruce Bagemihl's remarkable book exhaustively catalogues the immense variety of sexual behaviours observed throughout the entire animal kingdom in both males and females. Ranging from woodpeckers to sea lions, Bagemihl shows that animals of both sexes display varying degrees of male or female behaviour and have multiple shades of sexual orientation. In primates, too, especially in humans and bonobos (described below), Bagemihl notes that there has been a tendency to separate sex from reproduction, and to evolve various homosexual and non-procreative heterosexual activities.

The animal believed by some scientists to be closest to humans is the bonobo or pygmy chimpanzee, a small primate which was only discovered in 1929, when a German anatomist examining a "juvenile chimpanzee" skull realized he was actually looking at an adult skull belonging to a species of primate that hadn't been recognized before.

Scientists observed that about a third of bonobos mate face-to-face, a posture which before then was considered unique to humans.

·Another human-like feature in bonobos is that they have sex without regard to periods of fertility. Perhaps even more interesting, as Bagemihl reports, is that virtually all bonobos are bisexual: both the males and the females interact sexually with both sexes. Males commonly grab one another's penises in their hands and mouths, and among some females homosexual activity is. preferred over heterosexual. Bagemihl's book contains photographs of male bonobos engaging in fellatio and rump-rubbing, and manually stimulating the penises of younger males. Female pairs are shown engaging in genital rubbing, a behaviour not seen in other animal primates.

Most sex among bonobos appears to be just for pleasure, although they sometimes also use sex to smoothe over disagreements or to vie for a better position in the animals' hierarchy. Aggression is usually followed by sexual contact between the opponents, regardless of their sex; the sexual contact is thought to be the basis for reconciliation. Sex between females or between males serves as natural birth control. As sex is mostly unrelated to reproduction, females have only one offspring every five or six years.

Since the discovery of bonobos' sex lives, some sex therapists have begun promoting the "bonobo way of sex." Dr. Susan Block, who runs the Institute for the Erotic Arts and Sciences in Beverly Hills, has labelled bonobos "the horniest apes on earth." She encourages humans to follow their example in order to live in peace with one another. "Liberate your inner bonobo," she entreats. "You can't very well fight a war while you're having an orgasm." To translate her admiration for bonobos into action, she has pledged a share of the profits from her "ethical hedonism" TV and internet shows to bonobo conservation.

Bruce Bagemihl observes that sexual variations within species (including the human species) are the norm, rather than the exception, as are other kinds of variations — for example, variation in appearance or bodily form. He points out that genetic variation is essential for survival in all species. Instead of regarding variants in sexual behaviour as abnormal or undesirable, he urges us to see them as "an affirmation of life's vitality and infinite possibilities."

Applying his animal findings to humans, Bagemihl describes sexualities not simply as "male and female," but as "multiple" states. He describes gender as "kaleidoscopic" and sex itself as fluid (or multifaceted). This view of sex implies that there's a lot more to our sexuality than whom we choose to sleep with, a fact that has been noted by numerous observers. Psychiatrist Dr. Fritz Klein, who operates a private practice in San Diego, California, has argued that you can't describe a person's sexuality merely on the basis of whom he has sex with; you need to include factors such as sexual fantasy, sexual identity, and social and emotional preferences, and these factors may change over time. To address this problem, Dr. Klein designed the Klein Sexual Orientation Grid, which measures these various aspects in order to get a more complete picture of a person's sexuality. You can see what kind of picture of yourself emerges by completing the Sexual Orientation Quiz below.

❖ ——————————————————————————— ❖

SEXUAL ORIENTATION QUIZ

(adapted from the *Klein Sexual Orientation Grid*, by Fritz Klein, M.D.)

Look at the categories numbered 1 to 7 in scale 1 below. Then look at the table that follows scale 1 and scale 2. For each of the variables A to E, listed on the left side of the table, you must choose a category from scale 1 to describe your behaviour in three different conditions — in the past, in the present, and in your ideal future life. Write the three numbers for those categories opposite variables A to E. For variables F and G, choose numbers from scale 2.

"Past" refers to how you were prior to this year. "Present" refers to how you are now. "Ideal" refers to how you would like to be in the future, if you could choose.

It's not necessary to score this quiz; you can simply use it to get a clearer picture of the various aspects of your sexuality and how they may have changed over time. If you do want scores, total each of your past, present and ideal columns and divide each total by 7. Then compare your three averages to the numbers in Scale 2 and see which category your average number is closest to.

SCALE 1

1   Other sex only
2   Other sex mostly
3   Other sex somewhat more
4   Both sexes equally
5   Same sex somewhat more
6   Same sex mostly
7   Same sex only

SCALE 2

1   Heterosexual only
2   Heterosexual mostly
3   Heterosexual somewhat more
4   Straight and gay equally
5   Gay somewhat more
6   Gay mostly
7   Gay only

THE VARIABLES	PAST	PRESENT	IDEAL
A Who you're erotically attracted to			
B Who you have sex with			
C Who you fantasize about			
D Who you love and like the most			
E Who you choose to socialize with			
F What you define yourself as			
G Your lifestyle (openly gay, straight or bi)			

❖ ——————————————————— ❖

FIVE FACETS OF SEXUALITY

Were you surprised, when you completed the above quiz, that your own sexual orientation is more complex than you thought? And remember, sexual orientation is only one aspect of your sexuality. Think about the five facets of sexuality listed below, and you'll begin to get an idea of how diverse human sexuality actually is.

1   *Genetic sex:* which sex chromosomes you have. The most com-
    mon patterns are XX (female) and XY (male), but several other
    patterns also occur — for example, XXY (Klinefelter's Syndrome)†
    and XO (Turner's Syndrome)‡.

2   *Physical sex:* whether your genitals and interior sex organs are
    male, female or mixed. Usually a person's internal and external
    sex organs are consistent with one another, but sometimes they
    are opposite, or a mixture of the two.

3   *Sexual identity:* your internal sense of being a male or a female.

4   *Sexual orientation:* your primary erotic attraction — to males, to
    females or to both.

5   *Gender:* how you behave socially so that others perceive you as
    male, female or androgynous (having about equal amounts of
    male and female characteristics). That is, your talk, dress, ges-
    tures, walk, choice of activities and so on.

---

† *Klinefelter's Syndrome:* A chromosomal disorder in which one or more extra
x chromosomes are present. It occurs in about 1 in 700 male births. The usual pattern
is 47, XXY but infrequently it can also be XXXY, XXXXY or even XXXXXY. As the number
of xs increases, the likelihood and severity of mental retardation increases, as does the
number of genital and other malformations. Serum testosterone levels are low in
Klinefelter's males, who tend to have sparse facial and body hair and be hyposexual.

‡ *Turner's Syndrome:* A rare chromosomal disorder (about 1 in 2,500 female births)
in which the second sex chromosome is missing, so that the pattern is 45, XO. The
baby is born with female-appearing genitals and raised as a girl. Because there are no
fetal gonads, there is no onset of puberty and females are infertile. Males with
Turner's Syndrome have male-appearing bodies, a normal chromosome pattern and
decreased (though frequently normal) testicular function. Both females and males
with Turner's Syndrome are of short stature and display some or all of a number of
physical anomalies, including webbed neck, outward arm displacement, and heart
and kidney anomalies. In tests of mental abilities, Turner's female children and
adults do more poorly on tests in which normal females typically outperform men
than on tests in which males and females do equally well.

What complicates things is that these various aspects of our sexuality need not be consistent. Some people's chromosomes don't match their genitals. They may be genetically male but have female genitals, or vice versa. Other people's sexual identity is at odds with their physical sex. They have female bodies but feel like men, or male bodies but feel like women. Some people's sexual identity and physical sex are consistent but their sexual orientation is different from most others of their sex. Still others are born with sexual anomalies that make them difficult to classify.

Anne Fausto-Sterling, Professor of Biology and Women's Studies at Brown University, has calculated that for every 1,000 children born, 17 have some sexual variation in either chromosomes, hormones, genitals or gonads. That represents almost than half a million people in Canada, over a million in Britain and more than five million in the U.S. And those figures include only *observable* physical differences; they don't include the different erotic orientations or sexual identities, or the shades of maleness or femaleness. When you think of all the possible combinations of genes, hormones, physical body, identity, sexual attraction and shades of masculinity and femininity, you can see that it adds up to an incredible amount of sexual diversity.

Why isn't this more obvious? Because there are only two targets of erotic attraction — males and females. This gives the false impression that all the people who are attracted to one of those targets are the same, whereas in fact a variety of people with different sexual profiles can be attracted to the same target. You already know at least two kinds of people who are attracted to males — straight women and gay men. What is not so well understood is that those categories, "straight women" and "gay men" include a variety of subtypes, some more masculine than others, some whose sexuality differs in other ways. What if our sexuality were defined by our degree of psychological masculinity or femininity, or by some other aspect of our sexuality, instead of by whom we sleep with? Knowing only whether a person is attracted primarily to males or females tells us only one feature of the complete picture of that person's sexual life.

There's a lot more than that to be learned.

2

Sexing the Brain

Men are men, but Man is a woman.

R.K. CHESTERTON, *The Napoleon of Notting Hill*

GIVEN THAT WE LIVE nowadays in a sex-saturated environment, it's hard to imagine that for most of the world's existence, life was completely sexless. The tiny one-celled creatures that clung to life billions of years ago knew nothing about sexual reproduction; they simply reproduced themselves by cloning. A single parent made copies of herself, and the copy made copies of herself, and so on and on and on. Reproduction without the bother of sex. No heavy breathing or flimsy nighties snuggled against hairy chests.

But cloning had a big problem. It passed along to the next generation any chemical or radiation damage to a gene, and as the damage accumulated, it became increasingly difficult for offspring to survive. Small wonder then, that evolution pushed onward to something better. Over eons of time, more and more complex organisms gradually evolved, with various forms of reproduction, yet all of them still asexual. Until about a billion years ago, when sex finally entered the scene.

How it did, and why, are still mysteries, although it's generally recognized now that sexual reproduction does have a big advantage over asexual reproduction. Mixing the genes from two parents creates greater genetic diversity, and that leads to improved survival rates. This is true for all species, not just humans. In general, the more diverse a species is, the better its chances that at least some of its members will be different enough that they can adapt to any sudden change in the environment. If so, they could ensure the survival of their species that, without them, would simply have died out.

ADAM AND EVE REVISITED

It's now known that all of us descended from an "ancestral Eve" who's believed to have lived in Africa about 143,000 years ago. That finding by three American scientists created quite a media splash in 1987 when their study appeared in the prestigious science journal *Nature*. The scientists had discovered "Eve" by doing a worldwide survey of mitochondrial DNA, the DNA that resides in the cell's little powerhouse packages called mitochondria. Mitochondrial DNA has at least two interesting features: first, it's found only in females and, second, it passes down the maternal line without changing. Those features enabled scientists, by studying this DNA in women around the world, to conclude that all humans descended from a woman who probably lived in Africa about 200,000 years ago. That Eve, however, was an old-fashioned one: her genes needed about 57,000 more years to evolve into their *modern* form. That process was complete about 143,000 years ago, when our own "ancestral Eve" finally made her debut. As for Adam, you may be surprised to learn that his genes took 84,000 years longer than Eve's to evolve into their modern form. (I always had my doubts about that "Adam first, Eve second" scenario.)

Geneticist Peter Underhill of Stanford University discovered that modern man evolved a lot later than modern woman. Underhill's team studied Y chromosome markers in men from all over the world. (Only men have a Y sex chromosome; women have two Xs.) By examining the genetic variations they found in the Y, Underhill's group were able to trace back to our "ancestral Adam," who turned out to be a bushman living in Africa about 59,000 years ago.

Why the modern form of male genes took so much longer to emerge than those of female genes is another of those mysteries that science has yet to solve. Meanwhile, women may speculate that Mother Nature had to work a lot harder to produce an acceptable male. And men may argue that obviously it would take longer to turn out the superior sex!

Whatever the explanation, here we are for the past 59,000 years or so, two modern sexes reproducing ourselves by combining a female egg with a male sperm to form the genetic blueprint for a male or female offspring. But what decides which one it will be? If you remember this from your school biology class, just skip the next paragraph. If you don't, bear with me for a one-paragraph review.

Each body cell of a normal person has 23 pairs of chromosomes, and 22 of them are concerned with non-sexual aspects of development. They're numbered according to size: 1 is the biggest and 22 the smallest. Pair number 23 are the famous sex chromosomes; females carry two large identical Xs and males have one X and one small Y. The female donates to the egg one chromosome from each of her 22 pairs of chromosomes plus one of her Xs, and the male donates a sperm carrying one of each of his 22 pairs of chromosomes, plus either an X or a Y. The two kinds of sperm are produced in about equal numbers, so there's an almost equal probability of the baby being a boy or a girl. Once a sperm enters the egg and fertilizes it by combining its X or Y chromosome with the X in the egg, the fertilized egg will be either XX (a girl) or XY (a boy), depending on whether an X or a Y was the fertilizing sperm. The fertilized egg (called a zygote) develops into an embryo which, after several weeks, becomes a fetus which, after several months, becomes a baby.

Sounds so straightforward, doesn't it? So predictable. But any parents reading this know that it's actually an incredible process. I remember being amazed, when each of my own children was born, that somehow everything had worked out all the way from the fertilized egg to the fully formed baby. It seemed miraculous to me that all of the baby's bits and pieces were apparently in the correct amounts and in the right places. Oh, I knew the major events of fetal development all right, but I didn't know the details of that incredible process, nor the precise and orderly sequence in which they had to occur. I didn't fully appreciate that even tiny deviations from the timing of that sequence, or from the events themselves, could make a huge difference in a baby's development and eventual outcome.

I also had no idea, when a boy or girl baby joined our family, that its brain wouldn't be the same regardless of its sex. It had never occurred to me that there were "male brains" and "female brains," though I did begin to wonder when I saw how different little boys were from little girls. Initially, though, I attributed the differences to social influences. It was well known that parents didn't treat girls and boys the same; most people thought that was what made them behave differently. It wasn't until I became a psychologist and read the research suggesting that brains, like bodies, get masculinized or feminized in the womb, that I started realizing what was really going on.

BRAINS ARE NOT SEXUALLY NEUTRAL

A large body of animal research, and some human research, has now indicated that early sex hormones from the testicles and ovaries create permanently male and female brains. Exposure to androgens (male hormones) in the womb leads to a permanently male brain, which has male anatomy and produces typically male behaviours. For females it's ovarian estrogen that's responsible for feminizing the brain.

Once a human female's brain has become responsive to estrogen, shortly after birth, it continues to be so throughout life, causing transient changes in her brain and behaviour. If you're a woman reading this, you've probably been aware of mood changes that occur across your own menstrual cycle. Now recent studies have shown that it's not only mood that changes; changes also occur in the chemistry and even the *anatomy* of women's brains at different points in the cycle. As the hormones rise and fall across the menstrual cycle, the ebb and flow can actually alter the neural structure of a woman's brain.

These changes are only temporary, of course. But when sex hormones act on the developing brain early in life, they can cause permanent structural and biochemical changes, organizing the brain slightly differently in each sex. Boys and girls end up with brains wired to handle certain information differently, and to have different cognitive and emotional styles. Though their brains are also affected by learning and experience, those effects are believed to be limited by the biological constraints laid down in early brain development (more about this in Chapters 5, 6 and 7).

Overall, men's and women's brains are a lot more alike than they are different. Even under a microscope, the architecture of the male and female brain is very similar. And when differences do exist, they are average differences, telling nothing about any one individual. Having said all that, it's still true that there are observable differences between human male and female brains, just as there are in other animal brains. These differences are evident in the structure of the brain, in the way the brain is organized to process information, and in the different ways men and women sometimes think and solve problems.

STRUCTURAL AND FUNCTIONAL DIFFERENCES
BETWEEN MALE AND FEMALE BRAINS

What's the most obvious difference between men's and women's brains? Size. Male brains on average are about 15 percent larger than female brains, but nobody knows for certain what that signifies. It's well established that there's no difference in overall intelligence between the sexes, so brain size is obviously not related to that. Until quite recently it was believed men had larger brains because they had larger bodies, but that theory is now discredited because it's been shown that the relative brain size in the two sexes changes over the course of development. Until age two or three, brain size is actually about the same in both sexes. Then, as the brain grows larger, it grows more quickly in boys than in girls until age five or six, when the average boy has a larger brain than the average girl. By age five or six the brain has reached almost its full brain weight and, as boys and girls grow into adulthood, the difference in the size of their brains remains constant.

It may be that women's brains are laptop, whereas men's are desktop. A few years ago, Sandra Witelson of McMaster University reported finding that women's brain cells are packed more densely in a certain part of the cerebral cortex, that convoluted outer layer of the brain that looks like cauliflower but is actually grey matter composed of nerve cell bodies and their connections. (Turns out that women have 15 to 20 percent more grey matter than men.) Witelson found that the most tightly packed layers were the ones on the left that are linked to language competence and those on the right that are linked to the tonal, musical quality of speech. These findings may explain why females do better than males on a variety of speech and language tests.

Psychologist Ruben Gur, who directs the Brain Behavior Lab at the University of Pennsylvania, believes that the female's greater amount of grey matter gives her more concentrated information-processing power. In contrast, the larger male cranium is filled with more white matter and more cerebrospinal fluid (the clear fluid that surrounds and cushions the brain and spinal cord). The white matter, composed of the long tails of neurons, can broadcast signals throughout the brain, inhibiting the activation of other brain areas that could otherwise interfere with a current mental task. Gur believes this allows for the kind of "single-mindedness" needed to solve difficult spatial problems, at which men excel. As for men's extra cerebrospinal fluid, Gur believes men have more of this cushioning because they need it: they're more likely than men to get their heads banged about in fights or sports.

The greater density in women's cortices diminishes as they grow older and, coincidentally, become more prone than men to various kinds of dementia. Is post-menopausal loss of estrogen the culprit? Dr. Witelson thinks it might be, and that supplementation with estrogen might protect post-menopausal women from losing cortical cells. Other research, however, has suggested that supplemental estrogen, especially in high doses, increases the risk for Alzheimer's. Clearly, more research is needed.

Men also lose brain cells as they age, and more quickly than women. Between the late teens and the late 40s men's brain cells disappear almost three times as fast as women's, especially in the frontal lobes of the brain — the seat of higher-level mental functions including attention, planning, organizing, controlling impulses and applying social judgement. As the brain shrinks, the amount of fluid in the brain increases to fill the gap. Researchers measure the amount of fluid increase to see how much the brain has shrunk. What they've found, around the cortex, is a whopping sex difference: older men had an average 32 percent increase in brain fluid, whereas older women had only a 1 percent increase. In the front part of the brain, older men had an average fluid increase of 80 percent whereas older women had only a 37 percent increase. Laurence Whalley, author of *The Aging Brain*, suggests that the psychological changes typical of the elderly — shortened attention span, poor impulse control (including blurting out whatever's on your mind) and difficulty handling several things at once — may be due to shrinkage of the frontal lobes. Although as yet there is no accepted explanation for the lesser shrinkage in women's brains, it's been proposed that female brains may be protected by estrogen, at least until menopause.

Apart from size, male and female brains were, until the 1970s, believed to be identical. (I wasn't the only one who thought boys' and girls' brains were the same.) Then in 1975 neurologist J. A. Wada noted that a structure called the *planum temporale*, in the language centre of the brain, was shaped differently in men and women. In women it tended to be equal on both sides of the brain, whereas in men the left side tended to be larger, suggesting that men were relying more on their left brain for language. This finding was a great surprise, but soon other slight differences also began to be reported.

When scientists first reported these findings, they encountered a lot of criticism from feminists who were offended by the very idea that male and female brains might be different. Understandably, these women worried that a sex difference in the brain might be construed as "superior" vs. "inferior," leading to some predictably sexist conclusions. But science is neutral about its findings. If women are discriminated against because they're different from men, surely the solution is to abolish the discrimination, not to pretend they're the same. If we confuse equality with sameness, we should discriminate against people who are left-handed or extremely short or a different colour; those differences too are rooted in biology. It's one thing to believe strongly in equal rights for men and women (as I certainly do) but it's another thing to deny the scientific evidence that men and women are not the same.

Since the early findings of sex differences in the brain, evidence has continued to accumulate. After years of studying only dead brains, scientists in the last 30 years have been able to view living brains at work, thanks to the development of more sophisticated brain imaging equipment. This research has shown that male/

female differences are real, even after taking into account their difference in brain size. Some brain areas are larger in women and others larger in men. The sex differences appear only in certain areas of the brain and they're usually small. But even tiny structural differences can produce significant differences in thinking and behaviour.

Some of the more intriguing findings have been in the *hypothalamus* — a tiny, curved cluster of nerve cells the size of a thumb tip, lying deep in the front-centre of the brain. The hypothalamus acts like a pilot light for puberty, signalling the pituitary gland to tell the ovaries or testes to start producing sex hormones. It also regulates a number of bodily states, including temperature, hunger, thirst, sex drive and perhaps other aspects of sex. You may remember when the hypothalamus instantly became a star in 1991 after newspaper and magazine articles reported that a young neuroanatomist, Simon Levay, had discovered that its size differed in gay and straight men. (More about that in Chapter 5.)

The most conspicuous sex difference in the hypothalamus identified so far is a tiny area called the SDN (its real name is *the sexually dimorphic nucleus of the preoptic area*; you can see why it's abbreviated.) The SDN can be as much as two-and-a-half times larger in men than in women. It's important for developing sexual identity and behaviour, and it's extremely sensitive to sex hormones. Oddly enough, it's the same size in boys and girls until age two to four. Then, influenced by the different amounts of sex hormones they receive, it starts to shrink in little girls but not in little boys. Meanwhile, boys and girls are developing a male or female identity, an inward sense of being either a boy or a girl.

Some of our sensory organs also have sex differences. It's been known for some time that the *cochlea*, the spiral snail-shaped cavity of the inner ear, is more sensitive to soft sounds in women than in men. That's why a woman will hear every little snuffle the baby makes, while the baby's father sleeps soundly beside her. This sex difference in hearing is present in infants and children as well as in adults, which indicates that it's "hard-wired."

Another sensory organ, the VNO (vomeronasal organ, in the nose), is also functionally different in men and women. This organ is specialized for detecting pheromones — chemical signals released by one sex and evoking a response from the other sex. Women's VNO is especially sensitive to one particular male pheromone, while men's VNO is especially sensitive to a certain female pheromone. Like many other sex differences, the sex differences in smell are organized in the womb. You and I are quite unaware of the pheromones that influence us, because pheromones are *chemically* perceived signals, they're not *consciously* perceived as odours.

There's now some intriguing evidence that women are sexually attracted to men whose genes that code for disease detectors are different from theirs. These genes are known as "the major histocompatibility complex" (MHC), which is part of the immune system. Swiss zoologist Claus Wedekind discovered that a female mouse faced with different males will sniff their urine, which contains scented proteins identifying each male's unique set of MHC genes. The female will always choose the male whose MHC genes are least like hers. That's because his genes, when combined with hers, will give their offspring's immune system a wider variety of disease detectors. Wedekind extended the mouse research to college students, but asked the women to sniff men's sweaty T-shirts instead of their urine (for which I'm sure the women were immensely grateful!). Like female mice, women were most aroused by the scent of men with MHC genes different from their own — men whose genes, when mixed with theirs, would provide a greater range of disease detectors in their children.

New research has shown that the smell of men's armpit odours makes women feel more relaxed. The smell also triggers women to produce more luteinizing hormone, an important reproductive hormone.

RIGHT BRAIN/LEFT BRAIN — SEX DIFFERENCES

By now most people know that the two sides of the brain (called the cerebral hemispheres) tend to do different kinds of work. The discovery of this led to the publication of numerous books with titles such as *Left Brain, Right Brain* and *Use Both Sides of Your Brain*. Unfortunately, information in books of this type can be misleading. We do know some things about the two cerebral hemispheres (discussed below) but what's known so far won't enable you to analyze your personality or double your creativity. It's also important to keep in mind that *all* mental activities are actually whole-brain activities. It's not as though one side of your brain shuts down while the other side's working. But if you're involved in a mental task for which one side of your brain is more "talented," then that side will be doing the lion's share of the work while the other side does less.

The division of labour in the brain is called "lateralization," or hemispheric specialization. On average, men's brains are more lateralized — that is, more specialized for certain mental tasks — than women's. The male's left hemisphere tends to be distinctly better than his right for language-related tasks, and his right hemisphere tends to be much better than his left at spatial tasks. Women, on the other hand, tend to have hemispheres that are less specialized for these tasks. Their hemispheres tend to *share* in handling verbal and spatial tasks, rather than being separately specialized for each of them. That's why men and women often have different outcomes when they suffer a stroke.

If a woman has a stroke damaging *either* cerebral hemisphere, her scores on a vocabulary test are affected because both of her hemispheres are involved in language. In men, only damage to the *left* hemisphere affects their vocabulary score because that's the one primarily involved in language. A woman is also more likely to suffer speech impairment following a stroke that affects the front of the brain, whereas a man is more affected when the back of the brain is damaged. Similarly, in a woman the ability to initiate a desired movement of her hand relies on areas in the front of the brain, whereas in a man this ability relies on areas in the back of the brain.

When it comes to processing emotional information, a woman's right hemisphere is clearly the specialized one, but that hemisphere is much less specialized for processing spatial information, which is why women are better at handling emotional material than spatial material. In contrast, a man's right hemisphere is highly specialized for handling spatial information but it lacks the female's specialization for processing emotional information. As a result, men have a proven advantage in handling spatial information but are not as good as women in dealing with emotional information.

Scientists demonstrated this when they used PET scanning (positron emission tomography) to monitor men's and women's brains while they looked at pictures of actors' faces and judged the emotional expression on each face. Not only did the women's brains require less energy to interpret emotional expressions, but women were also better at determining whether the faces were sad. The men were just as good as the women at determining when faces were happy, however, so apparently they're good at happy but not at sad. (That suggests to me that, when a woman complains that her husband doesn't recognize when she's feeling down, she's telling the truth.)

Other researchers used MRIs (magnetic resonance imaging) to show that women's brains are better at feeling and recalling emotions. Men and women were presented with pictures of emotional scenes and then, three weeks later, they were retested to see how well they could recall the pictures. The results? Women's "feeling" brain was much more active than the men's when viewing the emotional scenes, and women were also significantly more accurate than men in recalling the emotional scenes. (One observer said the study supports the folkloric idea that a wife has a truer memory for marital spats.)

Women are also better at recognizing faces, say researchers at Sweden's Halmstad University. They recruited more than 1,800 men and women via e-mail to take part in a face-recognition study. Besides being more accurate than the men at recognizing faces, the women also were less distracted by details such as different hairstyles or changes in facial expression. In light of this, it was suggested that more women should be hired in security positions where it's important to be able to recognize faces in different contexts.

The sex differences in hemispheric specialization are present very early. At only three months of age, baby girls' and boys' brains respond differently to verbal and nonverbal sounds: girls show greater response from the left hemisphere and boys from the right hemisphere. As the left hemisphere is superior for language functions and the right for spatial functions, these very early responses appear to herald adult females' better verbal performance and adult males' better spatial performance.

But how do these sex differences come about? You probably won't be surprised to know that prenatal sex hormones set the stage for them. Researchers at the University of Waterloo demonstrated that very nicely. They measured the amount of testosterone in second trimester amniotic fluid (which had been obtained and frozen when expectant mothers had amniocentesis during pregnancy). When the children born to these mothers were 10 years old, the researchers tested them to see how their prenatal hormone level had influenced their hand preference and the way their brains' two hemispheres were specialized. They found that girls who'd been exposed to higher levels of testosterone in the womb than other girls were more strongly right-handed and had stronger left-hemisphere ability for speech, a pattern that's more often found in males. In the boys, those who'd been exposed to higher testosterone levels in the womb had stronger right-hemisphere specialization for emotion, a pattern more often found in females. For both girls and boys, then, the higher the level of testosterone in the womb, the more specialized each hemisphere became.

Other studies have shown that the two hemispheres mature at different rates in boys and girls. The right hemisphere matures earlier in boys, while the left hemisphere matures earlier in girls. The difference is established during the first year of life and continues throughout childhood development. It conditions how boys' and girls' brains will process information, and it influences what kinds of activities they'll choose and how skilful they'll be at various mental tasks and games. Because the right hemisphere of boys matures more quickly, they get a head start on right-brain skills, including spatial tasks such as measuring, map reading and mechanical design. In girls it's the left hemisphere that gets a head start, giving them an advantage in left-brain skills such as speaking, reading and writing. That's why, up to about age 10, girls tend to use verbal strategies to encode spatial information ("If I move the big block to the right of the small block, then it would look like …") whereas boys, instead of using words, use their specialized right hemisphere to mentally visualize this type of thing. But as the girls' right hemisphere matures, they begin, between the ages of 10 and 12, to use the right hemisphere for spatial information, as boys have been doing all along. However, because they've been slower than the boys in developing their right hemisphere, their spatial ability is generally not as good. Meanwhile, the boys have lagged behind the girls in left hemisphere development and consequently they are less skilled in the communicative aspects of language.

Of course environmental influences are also important in shaping how boys and girls think and solve problems. But scientists believe that the environment, from the beginning, is operating on brains that are already "wired" differently in boys and girls. It's not surprising then that in adulthood men and women tend to have different cognitive and emotional styles.

Simon Baron-Cohen, author of *The Essential Difference* (between the sexes) describes men as "systemizers" because they can intuitively figure out how things work, by extracting the underlying rules that govern the behaviour of a system. These skills require emotional detachment, so they're not much help in trying to understand *people*. To make sense of people requires attachment rather than detachment, and it's women who naturally attach. Baron-Cohen characterizes women as "empathizers" because they can spontaneously and naturally tune into others' feelings and thoughts, and it's that which makes real communication possible.

SEX DIFFERENCES IN COGNITIVE ABILITIES

When educators have measured school performance, boys have always been better at some school subjects and girls have been better at others. The differences between them have decreased over the years, probably because girls have received more encouragement in school and in society at large since the gradual mainstream acceptance of certain feminist ideals. But the differences in spatial and mathematical abilities are still there, especially at the highest levels, and high school girls still score lower in problem-solving tasks, despite the fact that nowadays girls are generally doing better than boys in school. At the annual summer Canada/USA Mathcamp for talented mathematics students from North America and elsewhere, boys typically outnumber girls five to one. On the other hand, the average girl today continues to show a clear advantage over boys in language skills and in emotional skills such as picking up on others' feelings and being able to "talk through" conflicts.

Such sex differences persist into adulthood. Of course there's always a lot of overlap between a bunch of men's scores and a bunch of women's scores. There are always women who do better than the average man in tasks where males excel, and there are always men who outscore the average woman in tasks where females excel. We're talking *group* differences here, not individual differences.

The two sexes sometimes use different strategies for solving the same problem — for example, how to remember a route. A woman will usually do it by memorizing landmarks along the way — the school, the drugstore, the neon sign (a strategy to which I personally subscribe), whereas a man (like my husband) will remember it more like a map. "Go north three blocks," he'll say, "then turn left and go west for about half a mile, and about 200 yards up watch the south side of the road for ..." but by then he's already lost me. I take comfort in the fact that I'm not alone in relying on landmarks: female rats also use them to remember how to run a maze. If a maze contains landmarks and the researcher removes them, the female rats will then get lost (as I would), while the male rats whip through the maze, unaffected by the missing landmarks.

In some mental tasks, men and women are equally proficient but they use different parts of their brain to do the job. Micheal Phillips at the University of Indiana found this when he compared the MRI results of men and women as they listened to a passage from a John Grisham novel being read. In all of the women, both sides of the brain were active, whereas in all but two of the men only the left side was active. Despite these different ways of processing the information, both sexes comprehended what they heard, showing that both mental strategies worked just fine.

Sometimes one mental strategy is better than another. A study in Germany suggested that men's superior spatial ability may be at least partly due to their brains using different strategies from women's. Men can navigate virtual mazes (three-dimensional computer mazes) more quickly and with fewer errors than women can. Knowing this, researchers in Germany asked men and women to navigate these mazes while their brain activity was recorded by an MRI machine. Men and women activated some of the same brain areas, but other areas were activated only in men or only in women. Apparently the two sexes were using different mental strategies to navigate the mazes and, as men were significantly faster at finding their way out of the maze, their strategies were obviously better.

Male rats are also better than females at navigating mazes, and it looks as though that's due to testosterone. Females become just as good as males if they're given a dose of testosterone very early in development. Early testosterone probably also accounted for the high spatial-ability scores in CAH girls (the girls in the last chapter who were exposed to abnormally high androgen levels in the womb).

But the most impressive evidence for the influence of sex hormones on cognitive abilities comes from Dutch studies of transsexuals who were given hormones to help them change into the opposite sex. Stephanie Van Goozen and her colleagues reported that female-to-male transsexuals, after being treated with testosterone, shifted from the female pattern of cognitive abilities to the male one — that is, their verbal fluency declined while their spatial ability improved. Exposing them to male hormone had made their brains as well as their bodies masculine. Just the opposite occurred with male-to-female transsexuals: after being treated with estrogen and anti-androgens, they shifted from the male pattern of cognitive performance to the female one — that is, their verbal skill improved and their spatial ability declined. Depriving them of male hormone and giving them female hormone had feminized not only their bodies, but their brains as well. These results provide some of the best evidence yet for a *causal* effect of sex hormones on brain functions. They also show that our brains remain susceptible to sex hormone effects even in adulthood.

Other studies have shown that fluctuating sex hormones can temporarily alter the cognitive performance of heterosexuals, too. Women perform differently at different points in the menstrual cycle (due to changing levels of estrogen and progesterone), whereas in men testosterone temporarily alters performance at different points in the day and in different seasons of the year. Doreen Kimura found that men's spatial performance was better in the spring, when their testosterone levels were lower. Elizabeth Hampson discovered that spatial ability in women fluctuated across the menstrual cycle and the changes correlated with estrogen level. When estrogen levels were low, women did better at spatial tests; when estrogen levels were high (just before menstruation), women did better in tests of fine manual skills and verbal skills. In other words, when a woman's female hormones were at a low ebb, certain of her cognitive skills were more like men's; when her female hormones were high, these skills were more stereotypically female. What's even more interesting is that not *all* mental skills were affected in this way, only those where there's a sex difference to begin with — for example, certain verbal and spatial skills. Mental tasks for which there's no difference between men and women were unaffected by changes in the sex hormones.

Geoff Sanders and Deborah Wenmoth at London Guildhall University wondered whether changing hormone levels might alter a woman's typical right or left hemisphere advantage for handling information. By testing women at different points in the menstrual cycle, the researchers learned that the usual left hemisphere activation for the verbal task was greater at the point in the cycle when estrogen was high, whereas the usual right hemisphere activation for recognizing musical chords was greater during menses, when estrogen was low. In other words, in women high estrogen is an advantage for tasks at which women normally excel (e.g., verbal tasks), but low estrogen is best for tasks in which men normally excel (e.g., music recognition).

But couldn't all the reported sex differences in cognitive abilities simply be due to adults' fluctuating hormone levels? Not according to research with young children, which shows that these differences originate in the sex hormone levels we experience in the womb. Researchers tested seven-year-old boys and girls on a spatial test called the "mental rotation" test, which required the children to mentally turn an object in space. Those girls who'd had higher testosterone levels in the womb (measured from their prenatal amniotic fluid, which had been frozen) were significantly faster in this test than other girls, whereas boys who'd had higher prenatal levels of testosterone were slower than other boys. Boys on average scored higher than girls on this test. But couldn't the boys' higher scores simply have been due to their having spent more time in spatial play? No, the researchers checked this and found that the amount of spatial play experience was not related to the child's mental rotation skill or to his prenatal testosterone levels. This study, therefore, showed that spatial ability is indeed determined by testosterone acting on the fetal brain. The study also showed that the same prenatal level of testosterone can affect each sex differently. Testosterone improved girls' spatial scores but lowered boys' spatial scores, just as later studies on adults showed that sex hormones can affect mental skills differently in men and women.

SEX DIFFERENCES IN COMMUNICATION AND RELATIONSHIP

Considering all the known differences between men's and women's brains and their cognitive abilities and styles, it's not surprising that they also have very different communication styles. Linguistics professor Deborah Tannen was the first to describe this in her two best-sellers, *That's Not What I Mean* and *You Just Don't Understand.* Tannen believes that women have a deep desire for intimacy while men have a deep desire for independence. This gives them different views of the same situations and also different talking styles. These in turn lead to "talking at cross-purposes" and getting into conflicts about dominance and control.

California psychologist John Gray followed up Tannen's research with his observation that the two sexes sometimes seem to be from different planets. In his hugely successful and entertaining book, *Men Are from Mars, Women Are from Venus,* Gray described how men and women "speak different languages," have different emotional needs and different ways of behaving in a relationship. Gray's assertions are supported by studies showing that women value empathy most in a friendship, whereas men value shared interests most. If their partner becomes involved in an affair, women tend to feel more threatened if the involvement is emotional whereas men tend to feel more threatened if it's sexual. Gray urged people, for the sake of peace, to stop expecting opposite-sex partners to be just like them and, instead, accept that the sexes are different and try to become more skilled at understanding where their partners are coming from. I agree with Gray's advice, but would add that each partner should have some good friends who could compensate in those areas where the spouse is not *simpatico*.

Some corporations are now hiring "gender relations specialists" to teach their male and female employees how to communicate more effectively with one another. One of those specialists is Barbara Annis, author of *Same Words, Different Language*. She points out that men and women problem-solve differently. Consequently, they react differently to a question like, "What do you think?" When a man hears that question, he believes he's being asked to make a decision, whereas a woman believes the question is asking her to explore the issue in an open-minded way. Not understanding that, says Annis, the man thinks the woman is muddled and unable to make a decision, whereas the woman thinks the man is trying to control her by shutting off discussion. Annis' advice is similar to that of Tannen's and Gray's: instead of criticizing the other sex, work at understanding where he or she is coming from when you're problem-solving together, and respond to that rather than to your own preconceived notions about the other sex. That's good advice, but you may need a therapist to help you actually put it into practice.

SEX DIFFERENCES IN BEHAVIOUR

Like other sex differences, differences in behaviour are quantitative, not qualitative. Men and women are capable of most of the same behaviours, but the likelihood that any particular one will occur differs between the sexes. In other words, they have different thresholds for doing, or not doing, a particular thing. The same is true for children: both boys and girls are capable of most of the same activities, but the *likelihood* of doing certain things differs between them.

Even in the womb there are sex differences: male fetuses are much more active than female fetuses. Is this a forecast of the rougher style of play that characterizes little boys? Probably; animal research has shown that higher prenatal testosterone does lead to more aggressiveness and rough-and-tumble play. If a male rat is castrated at birth, its play fighting is reduced to female-typical levels, whereas if female newborns are treated with testosterone, they can be induced to play fight at male-typical levels.

Newborn human infants also display sex differences. Researchers have found that girl babies are more sensitive to touch and sound than newborn boys, and more interested in human faces; they'll spend about twice as long as boys do looking at an adult face, and if the adult is speaking, they'll look even longer. In contrast, baby boys are typically not as interested in an adult's presence during the first few weeks of life; they also tend to be more active and more wakeful than girls the same age. In one study, one-year-old girls playing on the floor looked up at their mothers' faces significantly more often than the boy babies did. When the infants were shown a film of a talking head and a film of moving cars, the boys looked longer at the cars and the girls looked longer at the face.

Sex differences in play behaviour start to show up as early as 12 months of age. From then on throughout childhood, little boys on average show a greater preference than girls do for playing with vehicles, action toys and building materials. They tend to be more restless than girls, whose brains have higher levels of serotonin, the "calming" neurohormone. Boys also spend more time in play fighting and overall body contact. Their activities tend to be more competitive, whereas girls tend to be more cooperative. These sex differences are persistent. In adolescence and adulthood, and in a wide variety of different cultures, men are more physical and more physically aggressive than women.

Of course, not all men are aggressive and not all women are cooperative. We all know men who are gentle and women who are not. But individual examples don't alter the fact that, on average, men are much more physically aggressive than women, all over the world. Men commit many more crimes than women, and their crimes tend to be much more violent.

THE ROLE OF TESTOSTERONE

One of the biggest contributors to male aggression (though not the only one) is testosterone. Writing in the *New York Times Magazine*, Andrew Sullivan described the effects of the testosterone he injects into his body every two weeks. Sullivan is HIV positive, a condition that can cause muscle wasting and weight loss, which is why he began injecting testosterone a few years ago. Soon after injecting, when his testosterone level is at its peak, Sullivan feels "charged" — he gets a "deep surge of energy"; he needs to exercise more; his attention span shortens; his mind is faster, but his judgement is more impulsive; he's edgier and his anger flares more easily. Then, as the testosterone level starts to decline, Sullivan notices changes in his psyche and his behaviour. He becomes more garrulous and more social; his energy is redirected from action toward interaction. Sullivan describes talking to men in a testosterone therapy group; the men uniformly report that testosterone correlates with certain conditions — having energy, tenacity, strength, self-confidence, competitiveness and sexual drive.

Testosterone levels can temporarily rise and fall depending on the situation a person is in. As Sullivan explains, "Testosterone is usually elevated in response to confrontational situations — a street fight, a marital spat, a presidential debate — or in highly charged environments, like a strip bar or a pornographic Web site ... it can also be suddenly lowered by stress." For example, just before U.S. soldiers in Vietnam embarked on a fight mission, their testosterone levels dropped and remained low for a short time after the mission ended. Apparently stress affected their pituitary glands, which in turn lowered their testes' secretion of testosterone.

Becoming a father can also lower a man's testosterone. Biologists at Queen's University showed that, in first-time expectant fathers, the estrogen level goes up and the testosterone level goes down, compared to men who have no children. Perhaps the changes in expectant fathers' hormones help to "mellow" them, bringing out their nurturing and protective capacities in preparation for becoming parents. The same phenomenon occurs in mice, gerbils and hamsters that are new fathers. Similar drops in testosterone have been observed in men who settle into contented marriages.

As the last two studies showed, testosterone not only propels behaviour but responds to it — that is, it's a cause *and* an effect. Its level goes up in male tennis players winning a match, but *only* if the winning is very important to the player, and it goes down in losers. In men who don't regard winning the match as important, or who win by chance rather than by their own efforts, testosterone doesn't go up at all, or it goes up less. This pattern of responses is specific to men, possibly because (as several studies have shown) men are more interested in status-seeking than women, and dominating behaviour can enhance men's status (though not necessarily women's).

Note that it was a man's *feelings* about winning the tennis match that determined whether or not his testosterone level rose. The same effect of mental appraisal has been shown in rhesus monkeys. Testosterone levels measured before rhesus males were assembled into new all-male groups did not predict what rank a monkey would obtain in the dominance hierarchy. However, once the ranks were formed, the higher-ranking males developed higher testosterone levels. As with the tennis players, it was the *experience* of success or failure that altered the monkeys' hormone levels.

Certain occupations, including performers and trial lawyers, have been shown to correlate with high testosterone. Are high-testosterone people drawn to those occupations or does working in a "performance" setting encourage higher testosterone production? Probably both; as in the tennis game, testosterone both drives behaviour and responds to it.

Testosterone levels can be variable in women as well as in men. Female athletes have higher testosterone levels. Women who work outside the home tend to have higher levels than those who don't. Even the daughters of working women have been shown to have more testosterone than the daughters of stay-at-home moms. Are high-testosterone females more likely to seek work outside the home, or do their testosterone levels rise *because* of their outside involvement? At this point, nobody knows.

Testosterone influences aggression in women as well as in men. In particular, physical abuse among some couples has been identified as a significant problem in the lesbian community. I found in my clinical practice that, in every case where I treated a lesbian couple for spousal abuse, the abuse had been perpetrated by a "butch" lesbian against her "femme" partner. Butch lesbians have been shown to have higher levels of testosterone than femme lesbians. I believe this at least partly explains why they, like men, are more likely to perpetrate partner abuse than are others with less testosterone.

Some straight women also appear to be born with above-average testosterone levels. But although their levels are high compared to other women, they're still not comparable to men, and a woman with only average levels of testosterone probably secretes less of it than even the most timid man in the world (so long as he still has his gonads). Up to middle age, men on average produce 12 to 16 times more testosterone than women. After men are about 50, their testosterone levels drop and their ratio of testosterone to estrogen and progesterone gradually does a switch, so that older men end up actually having higher average levels of estrogen and progesterone than most women. This probably accounts for the tendency of most men to "mellow" as they age.

A friend of mine, father of six children, recently told me of his own experience with sex hormones after he learned that he had prostate cancer. Testosterone can encourage the growth of this kind of cancer and so my friend's treatment included giving him estrogen while reducing his body's testosterone. He tells me the treatment caused him to experience a profound change, not only in his libido, but also in his emotional functioning and even in his thinking. He's always been a good husband, but he says the estrogen treatments made it much easier for him to tune in to his wife's feelings and thoughts. His wife concurs with his opinion that, during this phase of her husband's treatment, they felt more like good women friends than like husband and wife. When the hormone treatments were stopped, my friend reverted to his old male self. He believes he may have to resume the estrogen treatments at some point, but next time he'll be prepared for his switch to pseudo-female.

PECULIAR PHYSICAL DIFFERENCES BETWEEN THE SEXES

Here's one you won't believe: men's body parts are larger on the right side and women's are larger on the left. Doreen Kimura found that men generally reported that their right foot and right testicle were larger than their left foot and testicle, while women tended to report that their left foot and left breast were larger than their right foot and breast. Even more surprising, Kimura found that being larger on one side or the other correlates with scores on mental ability tests. Both men and women with larger right sides did better on cognitive tests in which men usually excel, whereas the men and women with larger left sides did better on cognitive tests in which women usually excel.

Another interesting physical difference reported by Kimura and her colleagues was in the dermal ridges on the fingertips, those patterns that show up when people get fingerprinted. Fingertip ridges are developed in the fetus by the fourth month of pregnancy and remain unchanged throughout life. Men have more of them than women, and both sexes have more of them on the right hand than on the left. In the minority of people with more on the left, the person is usually female. What's more, incredible as it sounds, the number of fingertip ridges is related to people's mental abilities. People who have more ridges on the right do better than others on mental tasks in which men usually excel, and they do worse than others on mental tasks in which women excel. People with the opposite pattern —

more ridges on the left hand — have opposite results in tests of mental abilities. Recently researchers reported finding in children the same sex differences in fingertip characteristics, and the same associated cognitive skills, as in adults. (Fingertip ridges differ between straights and gays too, as we'll see in Chapter 5.)

It's not only finger*tips* that differ in the two sexes; the pattern of finger *lengths* also differs. Men typically have a shorter index finger than ring finger, whereas women usually have index and ring fingers about equal in length. The length of the fingers is determined early in gestation (before the 14th week) and testosterone is believed to be one of the major influences. From two years of age to adulthood, the sex difference in finger length remains unchanged.

But not all physical sex differences are caused by sex hormones. Men and women also have different *genes*, and this predisposes them to different health outcomes. As noted earlier, females have two x chromosomes, whereas males have only one. The female's two xs give her backup genes, so if a gene on the x chromosome breaks down, a backup gene can take over.[†] Men are not so lucky. If a man has a malfunctioning gene on his sole x chromosome, there's no backup x to help him out. That's why boys are more susceptible to a host of disorders linked to the x chromosome, including colour blindness and hemophilia (virtually all hemophiliacs are male.)

The male y chromosome isn't much help either, except for designing male embryos. Because it has only about 15 genes, the y

---

[†] It's not that every woman's cell has two xs; women undergo an early biochemical process that inactivates one x in about 81 percent of her cells. Sometimes it's the x donated by the father that gets inactivated and sometimes it's the x donated by the mother. But the 19 percent of xs that escape inactivation are still enough to provide backup genes. It's believed that the process of inactivating one of the female's xs may be what causes the higher occurrence of autoimmune disorders in women. For example, 90 percent of those with multiple sclerosis are women, and 75 percent of those with rheumatoid arthritis and lupus.

contains very little genetic information. Compared to the x chromosome, which has more than 1,000 genes and hence is rich in genetic
information that codes for a large number of traits, the y chromosome is a genetic desert. Desert or no, what makes the y invaluable is
one of its genes known as SRY, which starts the chain of events in a
developing fetus that makes its body male. Without SRY, a female
body would result because female is the default sex in humans and
in all other animals.

Geneticists have often wondered whether the poor y is on the
road to oblivion because it lacks a backup gene to take over when
damage occurs. Recently, however, a remarkable hidden talent in
the y was discovered. Unlike other chromosomes, it turns out that
the y has double copies of every gene encoded along it, one copy
written forward and the other written in the reverse. If a y gene is
damaged, the mirror-image folds itself over the damage and writes
over it, replacing the damaged letters of code with healthy ones. So it
looks as though the y is not headed for the dustbin after all; thankfully, about half of all babies will continue to be males.

Even when men and women have the same gene, it may be
expressed differently because they each produce different amounts
of hormones, and hormones are powerful regulators of genes. Certain genes may get expressed in only one sex or the other, or they
may get expressed at different times in men and women, leading to
different outcomes for the two sexes.

SEX DIFFERENCES IN HEALTH OUTCOMES

The Society for Women's Health Research (SWHR) in Washington,
D.C., has noted that scientists have known for a long time about the
anatomical differences between men and women but only in the
1990s did they recognize the significant biological and physiological
differences between the sexes. "Biomedical research has provided
evidence of biological differences between the sexes in virtually
every organ and system of the body and has resulted in the creation

of the field of scientific inquiry known as sex-based biology," reports the SWHR. One physician commented that doctors have practised medicine as though only a woman's breasts, uterus and ovaries made her unique, and as though her heart, brain and every other part of her body were identical to those of a man, which we now know is untrue.

The biological and physiological differences between women and men can produce dramatic differences in health outcomes. Here are some compiled by the SWHR:

- After consuming the same amount of alcohol, women have a higher blood alcohol content than men, even when allowing for size differences.
- Women who smoke are more likely to develop lung cancer than men who smoke the same number of cigarettes.
- Some pain medications are far more effective in relieving pain in women than in men.
- The same drug can cause different reactions and different side effects in women and men (even common drugs like antihistamines and antibiotics).
- Women have stronger immune systems than men, but are much more likely to get autoimmune diseases.
- Depression is two to three times more common in women than in men.
- Women's brains are less vulnerable than men's brains to aging effects, including less decrease in brain tissue mass.

In addition, it was recently learned that women are more susceptible to stress than men because their progesterone blocks the ability of the stress hormone system to turn itself off. Researchers discovered this by comparing men and women who were identical boy/girl twins, and learning that the females in these pairs were more affected by low levels of stress than their male twins were. As stress frequently leads to depression, this female susceptibility to stress very likely plays a part in the well-documented finding that women are at greater risk for depression.

SEX DIFFERENCES IN MATE SELECTION

For the past 70 years, psychologists have been asking men and women what characteristics they look for in a potential mate. Both have reported that they want mates who are intelligent, honest, loyal, kind, dependable and cooperative. But women always rated a partner's good financial prospects twice as highly as men. Newspaper personal ads reflected this difference: women listed financial security as a desired partner quality much more often than men did.

In the 1990s, psychologist David Buss surveyed more than 10,000 people in thirty-seven different cultures around the world. He found that in every case, women gave more importance to men's financial prospects than men gave to women's. Japanese women were the most interested in good financial prospects and Dutch women were the least interested but, even in the Dutch culture, women were more desirous of wealth in a potential partner than Dutch men were.

Buss also found that, in all the cultures he studied, women preferred male partners who were older than themselves. Men, on the other hand, invariably wanted younger women; they also valued physical beauty in women more highly than women valued it in men. In most cultures men also valued sexual faithfulness in women more than women did in men, but ironically, the men were still more likely than the women to seek sex outside of marriage!

But the times they are a-changin' — at least in the United States. Biologist Stephen Emlen at Cornell University recently reported his research findings that Americans nowadays want partners with qualities they value in themselves. Wealthy people want mates with money; handsome or beautiful people want mates who are attractive; people who want to create a family seek others like themselves; those who are ambitious seek ambitious partners, and so on. Emlen's research found that the desire for similar mates was five to six times stronger than men's desire for beauty or women's desire for wealth.

Other researchers have recently reported that many financially successful women are now choosing men younger than themselves, men who tend to have more "liberated" opinions about women than older men do. I believe that, as people become more and more psychologically sophisticated, they will increasingly tend to seek mates who are compatible rather than simply beautiful or rich. Mate selection is one sex difference that may, in fact, be disappearing.

3

Multiple Sexualities — The Majors

One half of the world cannot understand
the pleasures of the other.

JANE AUSTEN, *Emma*

S I WAS WRITING this book, people would
often ask me what it was about. When I told
them, their reaction was almost always one
of two kinds: either they were shocked, embarrassed and/or puzzled,
or else they were titillated and full of prurient interest. It occurred to
me that this dichotomy is typical of Western society's conflicted attitudes toward sex. On the one hand, obsessed with it, and on the
other hand, still not comfortable with it as a normal, natural part of
ordinary life. Advertisers skilfully play on that tension, using sex to
sell everything from cars to cough drops. The result is a social and
visual environment saturated with sexual images and innuendo,
which contributes nothing to a genuine understanding of human
sexuality and may actually work against it.

This chapter has a different agenda from that of the advertising industry. In attempting to familiarize readers with the sexual lives of straights and gays (our two major sexual categories), I hope not only to broaden understanding and acceptance, but also to increase readers' comfort with this normal, natural part of their own lives.

Heterosexuals

As everybody knows, heterosexuals are men and women whose genitals and sexual identity are typical for their sex, and whose primary erotic attraction is to the opposite sex. This is a convenient way to categorize people, but it's also misleading: "heterosexuality" is actually an umbrella term covering a variety of subtypes. All of these subtypes are attracted to the opposite sex, but their sexuality differs in other respects. As you read in Chapter 1, each of us has a sexual brain that's a unique combination of maleness and femaleness. Consequently, heterosexuals come in different shades, just as other sexual groups do.

Because heterosexuals are the majority, there's a tendency to think of them as "normal" and everybody else as "abnormal." But think about that: isn't it like saying that writing with your right hand is normal but writing with your left hand is abnormal, just because fewer people do it? Or that white skin is abnormal because the majority of people in the world have shades of brown or black skin instead of white? I think we should avoid the words "normal" and "abnormal" when talking about sexual types, and substitute words like majority/minority, typical/atypical, common/uncommon, usual/unusual. These words aren't judgmental. They describe minority types as just what they are — lesser in number — and they don't confuse big numbers with correctness. Belonging to a minority group doesn't mean you're abnormal, and being a member of the majority group doesn't guarantee that you're normal, either.

EROTIC ATTRACTION, NOT BEHAVIOUR

You'll notice that the definition of *heterosexual* here is based on people's primary erotic attraction. This doesn't mean that heterosexuals will never have same-sex relations, only that they will choose the opposite sex over their own sex whenever the former is available. In certain circumstances where the opposite sex is not available — for example, in prisons — heterosexuals will sometimes have sex with their own, but that doesn't change their basic erotic orientation. In his book *Palimpsest*, Gore Vidal describes frequent same-sex contacts among heterosexual men in the army during World War II, and even claims that on one Pacific island an entire marine division paired off. Presumably when these men returned home to their wives and families, however, most or all of them returned to exclusive heterosexual sex.

Surveys of prisons have reported that far more female than male inmates engage in homosexual activity, but most female inmates maintain a strong distinction between true lesbians who would prefer women outside of prison (and are therefore regarded by female inmates as "sick"), and women who merely "turn temporarily gay" while in prison.

Hispanic cultures in Central and South America and in the Mediterranean have also sometimes been cited as hotbeds of male homosexual activity. Sociologist John Gagnon at the State University of New York has observed that it's acceptable in those cultures for heterosexual men to engage homosexual men as secondary sexual partners. Men who do this don't see themselves as anything but heterosexual, and neither do their fellow citizens. That's because, in Latin cultures, so long as a man plays the dominant role in sex with another man, he is not regarded as homosexual.

The definition of *homosexual* in this book excludes the World War II men described by Gore Vidal, the Latin heterosexual men who sometimes engage in sex with other men, and the straight men and women who have same-sex liaisons in prison. If we were to measure sexual arousal in those groups, it would soon become obvious that they were not gay or bisexual, but heterosexual.

Since the 1950s, thanks to a Czechoslovakian sexologist named Kurt Freund, it has been possible to do such measurements on men (though only recently on women). Freund designed a device for measuring the increased erection of a man's penis when its owner engaged in sexual fantasy or viewed sexual pictures. The device is known as a "plethysmograph" (pleth-is-mo-graph). At first Freund used the device to try to change homosexuals' sexual orientation, but he found that that didn't work. Later he used it to classify male sexual responses. He found that heterosexual men's penises enlarged when the men were shown pictures of naked women but not when they were shown pictures of naked men or pictures of landscapes. Homosexual men's responses were the opposite: they got penile erections when viewing pictures of naked men but not when viewing pictures of naked women or landscapes.

Some of the men studied by Freund defined themselves as bisexual but in fact they were aroused only by erotic homosexual pictures and not by erotic heterosexual ones, indicating that they were actually homosexuals. Similar plethysmograph results have been obtained by other researchers. Sometimes men would deny that they were sexually aroused by certain love objects, but their enlarged penises would give them away. These studies showed that there are innate, physiological factors operating in sexual orientation. (More evidence for this in Chapter 6.)

SO WHAT DO HETEROSEXUALS DO?

It's surprising how little concrete information there is about heterosexual behaviour. Although nowadays we talk about sex *ad nauseam*, and a multitude of "helpers" issues nonstop advice about it, the scientific study of human sexual behaviour has tended to be seriously neglected and underfunded.

One of the few large surveys of sexual behaviour in North America, and the most recent, was carried out in the 1990s by a team of sociologists led by Edward O. Laumann at the University of Chicago. The survey almost didn't happen because the U.S. Senate, by a two-thirds majority, passed a law barring public funding of the study. Eventually the researchers were able to obtain private funding, but they still had to be extremely careful to word the questions so as not to make the interview "sexy or provocative or offensive." Later the authors would write, "Our study was completed only after a long and difficult struggle that shows if nothing else, why it has been so enormously difficult for any social scientists to get any reliable data on sexual practices."

Once they were able to get under way, the researchers, using a well-designed questionnaire, conducted personal interviews with a scientifically selected sample of over 3,400 American men and women aged 18 to 59 from across the country. People in the survey were asked questions about a wide range of sexual topics, including masturbation, sexual practices with partners, sexual fantasies and sexual preferences. Their responses to these questions yielded a massive amount of information. Here are some of the more interesting findings about heterosexuals:

The proportion of heterosexuals who had had five or more sex partners by age 30 depended on their age and sex. Thirty-eight percent of men in the oldest group, who grew up before the sexual revolution, reported that they had had five or more sex partners by age 30. In the younger group — men who had experienced the "sexual revolution" — that proportion was 49 percent, an increase of 11 percent. For women the increase was much more dramatic: only 2.6 percent of the older women reported having had five or more sex partners by age 30, whereas in the younger group that proportion was almost ninefold larger: 22.4 percent. It looks as though the sexual revolution in the U.S. was mainly a revolution for women!

About masturbation: more than half the women and more than a third of the men reported that they did not masturbate at all. The more educated people were, however, the more likely they were to report that they masturbated: 80 percent of men and 60 percent of women who had attended graduate school reported that they masturbated, compared to only 45 percent of men and 25 percent of women who had not finished high school.

About sexual techniques: 95 percent of the men and 97 percent of the women reported a lifetime practice of vaginal intercourse. A large majority of the heterosexual respondents did not practise anal sex, and those with a religious affiliation were even less likely to report its occurrence. As for oral sex, about three-quarters of both men and women reported having engaged in oral sex at least one time in their lives (again, the more education they had, the more likely they were to report this).

The study's authors commented on the dramatic increase in oral sex after the 1920s. "If there has been any basic change in the script for sex between women and men, it is the increase in the incidence and frequency of fellatio and cunnilingus." Among people born in the 1930s about 45 percent of women and 62 percent of men reported that they had either received or given oral sex at some time in their lives. For men born in the late 1940s, the incidence of "oral sex ever" had climbed to 90 percent; in women the trend peaked about a decade later at over 80 percent (women born in the late 1950s or early 1960s). However — and this may be a surprise to many people — only about a quarter of both men and women reported oral sex as a *current* practice, suggesting that most of these people had experimented with oral sex but it had not become a regular kind of sexual expression for them. Moreover, the youngest groups in the survey reported *lower* rates of oral sex than those born earlier, which could indicate either a current decline of interest in oral sex or, as the authors suggest, "these groups simply [may] have not yet engaged in sexual relationships in which oral sex has become likely ..." (My own impression, based on my clinical practice and various [non-scientific] magazine and television reports, is that the rates of oral sex have continued to increase in the years since the Chicago University data were gathered. In a recently published interview with high school students, girls as young as 13 reported that giving oral sex to boys was their preferred sexual activity because it enabled them to avoid pregnancy.)

Three-quarters of the men in the Chicago University study reported that they always have orgasm during sex with their partner, but surprisingly, only 29 percent of the women did so. Unlike the higher figures for better educated women in other areas of sexual activity, educated women were *less* likely to have frequent orgasm than were their less educated sisters. Women's lower rate of orgasm probably influenced the lower ratings they gave to "satisfaction with married sex." The researchers noted that the evolution of sexual equality in the 1960s and 1970s had created in women an expectation of mutual sexual fulfillment. If that wasn't occurring, women felt dissatisfied with the sexual relationship in their marriage.

There was a large disparity between men's and women's frequency of sexual fantasies and their use of erotic materials. More than half of the men, but only about a quarter of the women, reported fantasizing about sex every day or several times a day. Forty-one percent of men, compared to only 16 percent of women, made use of erotic materials including X-rated videos, magazines and books, sex toys, sex phone talk or strip clubs.

When men and women were asked to say which sexual practices they found "very appealing" males outnumbered females on every category, indicating that men generally find sex more appealing than women do. Nearly 80 percent of men and 77 percent of women endorsed vaginal intercourse as appealing. Almost half the men but only about a quarter of the women endorsed "watching partner undress" as appealing. A similar proportion of men and women endorsed "receiving oral sex" but only about a third of the men and a sixth of the women endorsed "giving oral sex" as very appealing.

One of the striking things about the above results is what they show about the differences between heterosexual men and women.

Despite the so-called "sexual revolution," this study clearly showed that men are still generally much more interested in things sexual than women are. This comes as no surprise to me as a psychologist, and probably to no other psychologist, either. In therapy with straight couples, "not enough sex" is almost always a male complaint, while "not enough romance and tenderness" is almost always a female complaint. Psychologist Roy Baumeister of Case Western Reserve University studied male and female sex drive and concluded that men's sexuality revolves around physical factors, in which biological nature tends to dominate and social and cultural influences are secondary. In women's sexuality, however, Baumeister concluded that education, religion and culture play the major role, while biological nature is secondary.

Isn't it a wonder that heterosexual men and women manage to remain paired despite their many sexual differences? And sex is not the only difference. As we saw in the last chapter, men and women differ in many other respects, too.

SWINGERS

In the decade of the 1950s a new social phenomenon called "wife-swapping" emerged in North America. Racy stories of husbands tossing their car keys into the middle of the carpet at the end of a party went 'round the suburbs. In choosing a set of keys, of course, a wife was also choosing someone else's husband to go home with that night. Eventually these stories faded; for a while it seemed as though the phenomenon had passed. But it proved only to have moved from the suburbs to the cities. Advertisements by married couples inviting other couples to "swing" with them began appearing with increasing frequency.

By 1960 more than a dozen magazines about swinging were available; soon they were advertising large swing parties in hotels and other venues. Then in 1969 a counselling psychologist named Robert McGinley opened a California club, called Wide World, for swinging couples. Armed with the contraceptive pill, women and their husbands joined other clubs that sprang up in cities and towns across the continent. In 1980 McGinley created an umbrella for such clubs, known as the North American Swing Club Association. Since then the subculture, later known as "The Lifestyle," has quietly and quickly mushroomed across North America.

Investigative reporter Terry Gould claims that "today in North America at least three million taxpayers in the 30- to 60-year-old age bracket are frequenting places where the opportunity to partake in open sexuality is the main drawing card." Gould spent a year studying the Lifestyles Organization and attending its gatherings. By the time he published his resulting book, *The Lifestyles*, in 1999, he was able to report:

> The lifestyle has grown so quickly in recent years that, wherever you live, you won't have trouble finding it ... It is a public, grass-roots, heterosexual orientation among mainstream couples who claim to have overcome the kind of loneliness, jealousy and shame adulterous marrieds endure. Lifestyle "playcouples" belong to three hundred formally affiliated clubs in two dozen countries, and to thousands of unaffiliated clubs ... Large lifestyle conventions are held 11 times a year in eight U.S. states, sometimes monopolizing entire resorts. The three-day Lifestyles '96 convention in San Diego drew 3,500 people from 437 cities in seven countries. One-third of the participants had postgraduate degrees; almost a third voted Republican; 40 percent considered themselves practicing Protestants, Catholics or Jews. Public figures with towering positions in society, pro-sex feminists, and even evangelical Christians attended the convention as "Lifestylers."

Gould reports that most couples in the Lifestyle are between 30 and 50 years old, and upper to middle-upper class. They are urged to practise safe sex, and condoms are conveniently available at parties and conventions. Partner-sharing is reportedly more common than "pile-on" orgies and, according to one of Gould's informants, a Lifestyle party doesn't always involve sexual intercourse among couples: "roughly 10 percent of the people who attend just like being in an atmosphere where such an interchange is conceivable." Some people reportedly practise "soft swinging," involving only nudity, massage and some sexual touching. Some people avoid "side-by-side" sex with another couple. "Open swingers" practice spouse exchange with the other couple in the same room. "Closed swingers" adjourn to separate rooms with their exchanged partners. "None of which," writes Gould, "is to say that on a roaring night I might not see wives involved in lesbian daisy chains three links long and other couples group-chambering the way I had seen the busy bodies at Vancouver Circles enjoying themselves."

Although the Lifestyle folks claim to advocate bisexuality in a spirit of sexual enlightenment, what they really advocate is bisexual activity for females only. Sexual contact between men is strictly forbidden (no rational explanation for this is proferred), indicating that the swinging lifestyle is prepared to swing in one direction only. This allows attendees to retain all of their prejudices about homosexuality and other sexual minorities. Their encouragement of same-sex activity among women appears to flow from the men's titillation when watching their women being sexually involved with other women. Although Lifestylers describe such sex as "lesbian sex," these women are firmly entrenched in heterosexual marriages, and I believe none of them would publicly call herself a lesbian. In fact, the swinging lifestyle is proudly defined as a heterosexual one.

(Some studies have shown that married women who have sex with women while staying married are not looking for alternate sex so much as they're seeking an emotional connectedness and friendship that's missing in their marriages.)

Typically it's the husbands who get the wives involved in swinging, but they claim that the wives, although initially reluctant, eventually become enthusiastic about it. Some women seem to be in it primarily for the culture and the socializing, but the sexual culture can reportedly also improve a woman's self-image. One woman told Gould, "This lifestyle is a way for women to get a feeling for being sexually attractive, i.e., 'I am more feminine and I am a more effective woman because these men want to have sex with me, and, therefore, I have power and an allure to my husband and to others.'" Another woman pointed out that middle-aged women in the Lifestyle can express their fantasies and begin to see themselves as "hot stuff." Gould says that many men in the culture see a healthy 50-year-old woman as more erotic than a 20-year-old because her sexuality is warm and frankly expressed.

In academic studies of swinging marriages, most of the women reported that they did not experience any same-sex fantasies or attractions before they became sexually involved with women at the instigation of their husbands or other swingers. However, after they had experienced pleasurable sex with other women, they did experience same-sex fantasies and attraction, though they emphasized that their primary attraction and sexual preference was still with men.

Despite the many pluses cited for the swinging culture, my own experience with swingers as patients tells me that the Lifestyle can be hazardous to marriage and family. The swinging wives who ended up in my office had usually begun the process by allowing their husbands to take nude photos of them. Later, they were persuaded to be photographed while being sexually involved with other women or men. Sometimes the husbands would get involved with other women (and occasionally with other men) too. Although the whole thing was supposed to be "just for fun," I have had cases, especially where the marriage is stale and/or lacking in emotional intimacy, where the "fun" ended up in a demand for divorce by one of the partners.

That's what happened with a couple I'll call Susan and Doug. Susan had become a "swinger" at her husband's instigation. She and Doug had two children. Doug liked to observe Susan being sexually involved with another woman, another man, or both. Usually Doug would photograph them; at times he would himself become involved with them. The couple came to see me after Susan told Doug she'd fallen in love with one of the male sex partners and wanted to leave her marriage. Though Susan was resentful that Doug had pressured her into these extramarital involvements, after a while she'd begun to enjoy the sessions with other men. She had initially disliked the idea of having sex with another woman, but eventually she'd been able to overcome her dislike, though she always preferred sex with men. Now, threatened with the dissolution of his family, Doug agreed to abandon the swinging lifestyle. Susan regained some of the power she felt she'd lost in their marriage, and consequently she began to feel less resentful and emotionally closer to Doug, which made it easier for her to give up the other man. Once she did so, she and Doug were able to focus on putting their marriage back on a more solid footing. They made good progress in therapy and were still together when I last heard of them.

Another hazard of swinging has been police raids on clubs. In 1992, 35 officers in bulletproof vests arrested 149 swingers inside Club Eros in Mississauga, Ontario, and charged them with being "found inside a common bawdy house." (They were later acquitted.) In 1998, when clubs in Montreal were raided, the police notified the press beforehand so that people could be photographed when they were forced into the street. It was five years before the Court's ruling came down. In July 2003, Judge Denis Boisvert ruled that the sex inside the Club Brigitte et Michel was "indecent" because police had testified that what they saw was an orgy taking place. The court concluded that "contemporary Canadian society tolerates swingers' clubs if the sexual exchanges take place in private. On the other hand, if the sexual exchanges take place in public … it does not constitute swinging, but orgies, and Canadians do not tolerate orgies." In 2005, however, swinging was legalized in Canada.

TRANSVESTITES

This is a subgroup of heterosexual men now commonly called "cross-dressers" because they enjoy dressing in female clothing. Like other heterosexual men, their primary erotic attraction is to women. Their only difference is that they become sexually aroused when they dress in female clothing, whereas other heterosexual men do not. When dressed as a woman, a transvestite *feels* like a woman, but at all other times he feels like a man. Cross-dressers enjoy having their wives watch them cross-dress and like making love to their wives while dressed in female garb.

Curiously, for some unknown reason, transvestism is limited to males. Heterosexual women apparently do not become sexually aroused by wearing men's clothing, perhaps because there are no rules against their doing so.

Some cross-dressers deny that they find cross-dressing sexually arousing, but a 1986 study by Ray Blanchard and his colleagues at the Clarke Institute of Psychiatry in Toronto suggests otherwise. Men were asked how often they had found cross-dressing to be erotically arousing during the past year. On the basis of their answers, they were divided into groups ranging from "always" to "never." Then the researchers measured penile blood volume as the cross-dressers listened to descriptions of cross-dressing and of sexually neutral activities. Regardless of which group the cross-dressers were in, their penises always responded more to descriptions of cross-dressing than to descriptions of neutral activities. This was not true of the non-cross-dressing heterosexual men in the study; *only* the cross-dressers found cross-dressing sexually arousing.

Some years ago a woman wrote to Ann Landers, then an American syndicated advice columnist, about cross-dressers: "… A cross-dresser can be your attorney, your physician, your child's kindergarten teacher or your druggist … they are sensitive, courageous men who are not afraid to express the caring, nurturing side of themselves. And … they are not gay." Landers received a large volume of mail in response to this letter and printed some of the responses in her March 17, 1997, column:

> My husband is the CEO of a Fortune 500 company. For the 15 years of our marriage, he has worn women's underwear. He is not gay. He enjoys the feel of it. We have a healthy sex life and two fine children. He told me his "secret" before we married, and it never made a difference to me.

> My husband is a cross-dresser, and I love it. When we take vacations, we dine in the finest restaurants, and he wears his fanciest outfits. I hate to admit it, but he is prettier than I am.

> People discuss cross-dressing as if it is playing "dress up." It is a lot more than that. It's a sexually fulfilling experience.

It's easy to confuse cross-dressers with transsexuals, who also like to dress as the opposite sex. But transsexuals feel like the opposite sex *all the time* and not just when they're dressing like women. (More about transsexuals later.) Cross-dressers also shouldn't be confused with straight men who dress as women strictly to get laughs. For example, Dame Edna Everage, the famous cross-dressing Australian comedian, is in real life a heterosexual man named Barry Humphries, who is married with children. Dame Edna gets laughs by exaggerating gender stereotypes. Wearing outrageous wigs, enormous eyeglasses and loads of jewellery, she likes to insult and humiliate public figures and other women. What distinguishes people like Dame Edna from transvestites is that Humphries doesn't become sexually aroused or feel like a woman when he's dressed as one, whereas transvestites do.

PARAPHILIACS

If you've ever been obsessively infatuated with someone, you may have some idea of how strongly attracted to a love object a paraphiliac feels, even though his love object is nothing like yours. The word "paraphilia" comes from para, meaning "beyond normal," and philia, meaning love. Thus paraphilia means "love that's beyond normal." The paraphiliac derives his sexual excitement and arousal from some bizarre imagery or act that most people wouldn't find the least bit exciting. Paraphilias are believed to originate in childhood and are very difficult to change in adulthood.

The majority of paraphiliacs are heterosexual males whose disorder manifests as a kind of addiction: the person is "addicted" to certain images or objects and is driven to respond to them erotically. A fetishist, for example, uses non-living objects for sexual excitement and arousal, often parts of clothing — a shoe, a sock, a scarf. In zoophilia, the erotic object is an animal; the animal may be trained to sexually excite the human by licking or rubbing. In voyeurism, the person needs to look at people (usually strangers) naked or undressing. These "peeping Toms" do not attempt to have sexual contact with the people they spy on; it's the looking that arouses them.

A 34-year-old patient of mine suffered from a paraphilia known as exhibitionism. Married and the father of two young boys, Ron (not his real name) was driven to expose his genitals to girls and women in parks and other public places. He was an emotionally immature man whose wife complained that he often experienced sexual difficulties in their marriage, but otherwise he was a good husband and father. Ron had managed to escape detection from both the police and his wife until two things happened in the same week. His wife discovered, at the back of his closet, a coat with two pant legs suspended from the lining so that when the coat was closed, Ron would appear to be fully clothed under it. When the coat was unbuttoned, he would be naked where the rest of the pants should have been. When the outfit was discovered by his wife, Ron passed it off as a spoof he was preparing for an upcoming office party. Then, two days later, he was arrested for exposing himself outside the women's washroom at a local shopping mall.

The combination of these two events, along with his wife's threats of leaving him and taking the children, motivated Ron to seek treatment. As he had never been in trouble with the law before, he was put on probation. I saw him regularly for several months, alone and with his wife, and he made good progress. At follow-up nine months later, he was still doing well, though that was no guarantee that he would not reoffend sometime in the future.

Sexologist John Money, author of *Gay, Straight and In-Between*, gives examples of other paraphilias that are even more unusual. One of these involved a professor of architectural design engineering who, from the age of 13, was obsessed with the desire to have his leg amputated above the knee. Since then, the image of himself as an amputee had been an erotic fantasy that accompanied every sexual experience of his life. Over several years, he'd undergone long periods of psychotherapy, to no avail. He had also tried to make himself an amputee by drilling into his own leg, but this, too, failed. Money speculated that this man desired to win his father's approval by becoming his daughter; as he was reluctant to sacrifice his penis to this cause, he wished to sacrifice his leg instead. (Don't try to make sense of this, it's a disorder.)

Another man described by Money had asphyxiophilia (literally "in love with asphyxiation"). He substituted for his own asphyxiation the images of women in horror films or on television, drowning or being choked to death. These scenes were extremely erotic for him: while watching, he would masturbate to orgasm. He claimed to have had this condition since about age 10 and wanted to be rid of it.

There are a lot of other paraphilias, most of which, though bizarre, are no threat to other people. Several paraphilias, however — including Ron's exhibitionism described above — are forbidden by law. The best known one, and undoubtedly the most generally loathed, is pedophilia. For a pedophile, the act or fantasy of having sex with children is the preferred or exclusive method of achieving sexual excitement. There's a popular misconception that most pedophiles are homosexual. In fact, most pedophiles are hetero-sexual men who are married or have been married. Their prefer-ence, which is for eight- to 10-year-old girls, usually manifests itself in middle age. The minority of pedophiles who are homosexual prefer slightly older boys.

What about the other colours in the heterosexual rainbow that have not yet been described? If we're going to learn more about those, we'll need to start providing much more public funding for scientific research into human sexuality than we've seen so far. Although some aspects of sexuality have been studied in various select groups, the sex life of the general population has been largely ignored by public health ministries. There were no major follow-up studies of the famous Kinsey reports (of which more later) for almost four decades, when the 1994 Chicago University survey (cited ear-lier) was done. But that study almost didn't get done; it was denied public funding and was only made possible by the eventual support of several private foundations.

Homosexuals

These are men and women with genitals typical for their sex, who identify inwardly as male or female in accordance with their geni-tals, and whose primary erotic attraction is to their own sex.

Same-sex behaviour occurs for other reasons, too, but the people involved are not homosexual. For example, in certain cultures same-sex behaviour has been a ritual for all boys as part of their develop-ment into adults, but the boys were almost invariably heterosexual as adults. Among the Sambia, a small isolated tribe in the New Guinea highlands, boys were required to fellate the youths of the tribe because of a cultural belief that boys would only become real men if they swallowed semen. Both the boys and the youths were taught that female bodies were poisonously dangerous for them. Despite such conditioning, almost all Sambian men were heterosexual. In adulthood, fellatio was not allowed (that would be stealing semen needed by the younger boys); men acquired wives and settled into family life. When an occasional Sambian man proved to be truly homosexual — erotically attracted only to men — his behaviour was incomprehensible to other Sambians. (The Sambians' ritual same-sex behaviour in boys was stopped in the 1980s by the intervention of missionaries.)

In another New Guinea culture, the Kaluli, anal intercourse was used to transmit semen from older men to younger boys, for the purpose of making the boys into men. Again, almost all of these boys became exclusively heterosexual when they matured. They also reported that heterosexuality in adulthood was their preference, indicating that their shift was not socially induced.

Same-sex behaviour in the Sambians and Kaluli did not represent a homosexual orientation; it was merely part of an enforced tribal ritual during a limited period of time in males' lives. In what follows, we will be looking at men and women for whom same-sex behaviour arises spontaneously. They prefer to have sex with same-sex partners because that's who they are erotically attracted to.

HOMOSEXUALITY IS WORLDWIDE

Several studies have shown that homosexuality occurs all over the world. Half a century ago anthropologist C. S. Ford and psychologist F. A. Beach studied 76 diverse societies around the world. They found that in almost two-thirds of these societies homosexual activities were considered either normal or socially acceptable, at least for certain members of the community. Even in some of those societies that condemned or prohibited homosexual practices, they still took place secretly.

In North America, aboriginals who were not heterosexual were named "berdache" by 18th Century French anthropologists who thought these people represented a new form of sexual variance. Since then the berdache have been extensively written about, often as some kind of "third sex." More recently, however, it has been learned that the berdache were actually a mixed group that included homosexuals, transvestites, transsexuals and intersexuals — some of the same types of sexual variants as occur in contemporary society.

Male Homosexuality in Four Societies, an interesting book written in 1985 by sociologists Frederick Whitham and Robin Mathy, reported the results of their survey of homosexual men in Brazil, Guatemala, the Philippines and the U.S. (Arizona and Hawaii). Some of these societies are tolerant of homosexuality, while others are highly intolerant. Nonetheless, homosexuality occurred with equal frequency in the various cultures, regardless of whether that culture was tolerant or hostile. The researchers identified three types of homosexual men: about 10 percent had no early feminine behaviour and were quite masculine adults; about 65 percent had some "girlish" behaviour in childhood but at puberty were masculinized; about 25 percent showed extensive "girlish" behaviour as children and as adults were quite effeminate. The researchers found no evidence that family factors determined sexual orientation in any of the cultures studied.

In 1998 Whitham and a group of researchers from Arizona State University published questionnaire data obtained from lesbian and heterosexual women in Brazil, Peru, the Philippines and the U.S. between 1981 and 1988. They found that a population of lesbian women was always present and there were similarities in the development of lesbian sexuality, regardless of culture. Some cultures attempted to suppress emerging lesbian behaviour in girls, but they generally succeeded only in impeding its development rather than obliterating it. Usually lesbian orientation would eventually overcome the attempts to suppress it, regardless of the kind of society in which these young women were raised.

HOW MANY HOMOSEXUALS ARE THERE?

The answer to that question depends on who you talk to. Estimates in the U.S., Canada and Europe have varied widely from 10 percent

(Kinsey) to more recent figures of two to three percent for men and about half that number for women. Part of the problem, as with other estimates of sexual types, has been the lack of reliable and objective research. Until fairly recently, homosexuality in Western countries was widely viewed as a perversion, a sin or a mental disease. Consequently, people were reluctant to label themselves as homosexual or even to admit to researchers that they engaged in same-sex behaviour.

One of the earliest attempts at a widescale study of homosexuality in the U.S. was by biologist Alfred Kinsey of Indiana University, a trailblazer in the field of sexology. Using a seven-point scale ranging from "exclusively heterosexual" to "exclusively homosexual," the Kinsey researchers interviewed thousands of American men and women about their sexual feelings and behaviours, rated them and published the results in two large reports, *Sexual Behavior in the Human Male* (1948) and *Sexual Behavior in the Human Female* (1953).

The popularity of Kinsey's reports surprised everyone. The publishers had originally planned to print 10,000 copies; amazingly, 200,000 copies sold in the first six months. Public reaction to the 1948 report on males was largely positive, although many people were shocked (or titillated) to learn how many men had been sexually involved with women other than their wives or (even worse!) with other men. Even so, negative reaction to the 1953 report on females was much stronger. The report caused such public furor, in fact, that the Rockefeller Foundation terminated its funding for Kinsey's research. Obviously the American public was not ready to hear about women having sex outside the sanctity of marriage, or even within the bonds of marriage but beyond the missionary position. But the genie was out of the bottle. Kinsey had opened the way for public discussion of a range of sexualities and a variety of sexual practices. The lid would never be put back on the bottle again.

Kinsey reported that four percent of the men he interviewed and two percent of the women were exclusively homosexual throughout their lives. He also reported that 10 percent of the males were "more or less" exclusively homosexual for at least three years between the ages of 16 and 55. Unfortunately, the 10 percent figure was seized upon in some quarters as an accurate estimate of the prevalence of homosexuality, an error that persisted for many years.

Thirty-seven percent of Kinsey's male population reported that they'd had at least one homosexual encounter in their lives. However, when other researchers later analyzed Kinsey's data, they found that a high proportion of these men had their homosexual experience in adolescence or earlier, and not in adulthood. For most of them, homosexual activity was probably due to adolescent "crushes" or experimentation rather than to true sexual identity.

A surprising finding in the 1948 Kinsey study was that homosexual males did not fit the old stereotype of homosexuals as people constantly engaged in sexual activity. In fact, the gay men in Kinsey's study actually had fewer sexual contacts than the straight men did, a finding that was confirmed in a 1960 study.

Kinsey's studies were landmarks in the study of human sexuality, but they suffered from serious problems in design and methodology. People who took part in the studies were all volunteers instead of being recruited by scientific sampling, which meant that the results could not be generalized to a wider population. Also, instead of administering the interview questionnaire in the same way to all respondents, Kinsey's interviewers were allowed to vary the order and the wording of their questions, which could have skewed the answers. In addition, responses to his seven-point scale were sometimes questionably interpreted. For example, when counting homosexual contacts Kinsey included *all* physical contacts, even nonsexual ones, such as girls dancing together; this was bound to inflate his figures for homosexual activity. Despite these shortcomings, however, Kinsey's work is still highly valued because his groundbreaking studies paved the way for future inquiries into human sexuality.

Twenty years after Kinsey's reports, a team led by Alan Bell and Martin Weinberg of Indiana University conducted lengthy telephone interviews with almost a thousand homosexual men and women in the San Francisco Bay area. These were compared to a heterosexual group comparable in age and education. Among the homosexual adults surveyed, the researchers found a wide diversity of feelings, behaviours, dreams and fantasies. The title of their book *Homosexualities* reflected their view that there is no single type of homosexual person; there are numerous ways to be homosexual and to express one's homosexuality.

The majority of the men in this study reported having sex with other men at least twice a week, while nearly half of the women reported having sex with other women less than once a week. The researchers observed that, in general, males (gay or straight) tend to be more sexually driven than females. Females tend to de-emphasize the sexual features of their relationships and emphasize other aspects. (More about this later.)

Bell and Weinberg divided their homosexual subjects into five groups. Lesbian and gay couples in the "close-coupled" group were similar to happily married heterosexual people. (Some of them even described themselves as "happily married.") Partners in this group were closely bound together and their partnerships tended to be the source of all of their sexual and interpersonal satisfactions. These individuals had the smallest number of sexual problems and were the least likely to regret that they were homosexual. They preferred to spend their evenings at home together. Their psychological adjustment was generally very good. They were happier than any of the other groups; in fact, the lesbians in this group were the least likely of all the groups ever to have felt the need to seek professional counselling for a personal problem.

People in the second group — the "open-coupled" — were also living with sexual partners, but unlike the "close-coupled" groups, they were unhappy with their relationships and tended to seek satisfaction with people other than their partners. The men did more cruising than average, and the lesbians in this group cruised more than any of the lesbians in the other groups. Psychologically, people in this group were average, compared to all of the other respondents, but the men were more self-accepting and less lonely than the women.

People in the "functionals" group tended to be the "swinging singles" whose lives were organized around their sexual experiences. They cruised frequently, were the most interested in sex of all the groups, and had had more partners than any of the others. Nonetheless, their psychological adjustment was quite good: they tended to be energetic and self-reliant, cheerful and optimistic, and comfortable with their emphasis on sex. They had few sexual problems but, although they were were not generally depressed or unhappy, they were still not as happy as the "close-coupled" people.

The fourth group were the "dysfunctionals" — people who could be described as the stereotypically "tormented homosexuals." These were troubled people whose sexual, social and psychological adjustments were poorer than all of the other groups. They had the most sexual problems and generally regretted being homosexual. They tended to think of themselves as sexually unappealing and had the most difficulty in finding partners. The men in this group had suffered the most in terms of having been assaulted or having had job problems due to their sexual orientation. Lesbians in this group were the most likely to have needed long-term professional help for their problems.

The researchers noted that if they had seen only the "dysfunctional" group of homosexuals, they would have (erroneously) concluded that homosexuals are men and women who are "conflict-ridden social misfits." In fact, in terms of social and psychological adjustment, most of the other homosexuals in the survey were indistinguishable from the heterosexuals, except that they were less self-accepting and experienced more loneliness and depression. These feelings may well have been a normal reaction to the extreme degree of prejudice directed against homosexuals at that time. The researchers pointed out that "dysfunctionals" also existed within the heterosexual population.

The last group were the "asexuals," who tended to be loners. They reported less interest in sex, few partners and a poor opinion of their own sex appeal. Not surprisingly, people in this group tended to have sexual problems.

Bell and Weinberg's survey was limited to the San Francisco Bay area and the people who took part in it were not recruited scientifically. It was not until the publication of the big 1994 study by the University of Chicago team, described previously, that reliable numbers for homosexuals in the entire U.S. were available. In that study, only 2.8 percent of the men and 1.4 percent of the women identified themselves as homosexual or bisexual, though a much higher number reported that they had experienced same-sex *desire* (7.7 percent percent of the men and 7.5 percent of the women), or same-sex *behaviour* (7.1 percent of the men and 3.8 percent of the women.) Almost half of the men who reported ever having had sex with another man had done so before they turned 18 and not after that. This is consistent with Kinsey's finding that many men who at some time had sex with another man did so in adolescence or earlier, but not in adulthood.

An interesting finding in the University of Chicago study was the difference between the number of gay men living in big cities and those living in other parts of the country. In the 12 largest metropolitan areas of the U.S., men reported rates of homosexuality between 9.2 percent and 16.7 percent. A similar concentration of gay men in London was reported in a 1992 British study by Anne Johnson and colleagues. In both the U.S. and Britain, the population rates of homosexuals were highest in densely populated areas and declined as the population density diminished. Either homosexuals tend to be born in cities, or more likely, they congregate there because cities provide a more congenial environment for them. (Recently some lesbian and gay writers have described their own positive experience of living in small towns and rural communities, and urged others to do the same. The hope is that, as rural people finally get to know gay and lesbian people as their neighbours, dealing with the same things that straight rural people deal with on a daily basis, they will become more accepting of homosexuality.)

As for the women in the University of Chicago study, their rates for same-sex involvement were always lower than they were for men, although more women than men reported that they found the notion of same-sex *appealing*. Education was a more important factor in female same-sex involvement. Women who had graduated from college always reported the highest level of homosexual involvement, whereas women with high school education or less reported very low rates of such involvement. Similarly, male college graduates were twice as likely to be gay or bisexual as male high school graduates. (This doesn't mean that going to college caused them to be gay; instead, it's likely that being gay made them more interested in college.)

The average frequency of sex for gay men with partners was slightly lower than the average for straight men with partners, but the rates for gay and straight women hardly differed. As for homosexual sexual practices, the rate of masturbation was almost three times higher in homosexuals than in the total survey group; oral sex was almost universal in both men and women; anal sex among the homosexual men was less common than oral sex, but more common than for heterosexuals.

The 2.8 percent and 1.4 percent figures for male and female homosexuals in this study are fairly similar to rates reported in two European surveys. In a large 1993 French survey 1.1 percent of men reported having had sex with another man during the past year and another 3 percent reported having had any male sex partners in their entire lives. In Britain's first large national survey of sexual behaviour in 1992, 1.1 percent of men reported same-sex experience in the past year and 3.6 percent reported some same-sex experience ever. None of the figures reported in these three large studies come anywhere near the 10 percent figure for male homosexuality that was based on Kinsey's report that 10 percent of American men were "more or less" exclusively homosexual. In 1997 Scott Hershberger at the University of Kansas surveyed twins from the Minnesota Twin Registry and reported that the prevalence of homosexuality was 2.5 percent for men and 1.68 percent for women. In 2000, a group of American pub-· lic health researchers who analyzed responses in a large national survey of twins reported identical rates for male homosexuality as those in the big University of Chicago study, and slightly lower rates for female homosexuality — that is, 3.1 percent for men and 1.5 percent for women.

Considering all these figures together, it appears that two to three percent of men and about one to two percent of women are homosexual. Those are small percentages, but they represent a very large number of people. In the U.S., for example, based on the above per-centages, there could be more than three million people age 20 and over who are gay. In Britain the number may be up to 650,000, in Canada more than 300,000. In the entire world there must be somewhere between 37 and 56 million men and between 19 and 37 million women who are gay. Added together, their numbers could well exceed the entire population of Germany, be equal to about one-third of the entire population of the United States and be three times the population of Canada. These are estimates, of course, but they show that small percentages can be very misleading. And even these large numbers are probably underestimates, as they're based on self-report. I think it's highly likely that many people were reluctant to identify themselves as homosexual, either for fear of disapproval or because they hadn't yet admitted to themselves that they were gay.

DIFFERENT TYPES OF HOMOSEXUALITY

Virtually all sexologists nowadays agree that there are several different types of homosexuality, but the classification of types differs from one researcher to another. In the Bell and Weinberg survey cited earlier, homosexuals were grouped according to their lifestyles. In 1987 James Weinrich, an evolutionary biologist and sexologist at the University of California at San Diego, proposed a model classifying different kinds of homosexuals, bisexuals and transsexuals according to their degree of masculinization and feminization.

A variety of psychological tests have been administered to homosexual men and women over the years to determine their degree of femininity or masculinity. In virtually all of these tests, gay men averaged higher feminine scores than straight men, and lesbians averaged higher masculine scores than straight women. However, on more recent sex role inventories that treat masculinity and femininity as independent traits (instead of being on a continuum), very often gay men score just as masculine as straight men, and lesbian women score just as feminine as heterosexual women. This shows there are two things going on: the average gay man is more feminine than straight men, but not less masculine. Similarly, the average lesbian is more masculine than her straight sisters, but not less feminine. "Average," of course, covers a wide range; there are gay men who aren't feminine at all, and lesbians who are more feminine than most straight women.

Do gays and lesbians typically prefer masculine or feminine partners? To find out, psychologist Michael Bailey and his colleagues at Northwestern University examined personal ads placed by gays and lesbians seeking partners. The researchers found that the average gay man preferred men who described themselves as masculine rather than feminine, but this preference was weaker among men who rated themselves as relatively feminine. Lesbians preferred women who described themselves as feminine-looking, but did not discriminate against women calling themselves masculine.

Jim McKnight, chair of the Psychology Department at the University of Western Sydney, has proposed a typology for gay men that has nothing to do with being masculine or feminine. McKnight's groups are called the Experimenters, the Swingers, the Unwanted, the Predisposed and the Driven. According to McKnight, Experimenters are adolescents (and some adults) who engage in homosexual behaviour out of curiosity rather than innate orientation; some Experimenters may "like what they find and decide to stay." McKnight's Swingers engage in sex with both men and women, sometimes from a heightened sex drive. These men may be homosexual, bisexual or heterosexual. The Unwanted, according to McKnight, are men who are unable to get heterosexual partners and so fall back on homosexuality as a "second-best" option. The Predisposed are described as men who knew they were gay from adolescence or earlier. These men, suggests McKnight, may be biologically predestined to be gay. And finally, the Driven are men described by McKnight as feeling compelled to express their homosexuality despite internalized homophobia and social disapproval. McKnight proposes that in these men homosexuality is a consequence of a "dose-dependent mix of genes." It's anybody's guess at this point whether any of these categories is valid or whether they're just convenient labels for thinking about people's differences. Like a lot of other things in this field, more research is needed.

ARE GAY MEN OVERSEXED?

Surveys of gay men in the San Francisco area — after large numbers of them had come out of the closet and before the AIDS epidemic appeared — reported very large numbers of sexual partners, frequently 100 or more. (This was not true of gay women in the area.) The practice of anonymous gay sex in parks and public baths was cited as evidence that gay men are oversexed. Several observers have argued, however, that these gay men were simply being male, unrestrained by the limitations normally set by female partners in heterosexual encounters. Anthropologist Donald Symons writes, "I am suggesting that heterosexual men would be as likely as homosexual men to have sex most often with strangers, to participate in anonymous orgies in public baths and to stop off in public restrooms for five minutes of fellatio on the way home from work if women were interested in these activities. But women are not interested."

A Bradley University study of more than 16,000 people around the world found that men everywhere want more sexual partners than women do. But "want" and "get" are two different things. Donald Symons comments that every heterosexual relationship is a compromise between the wants of a man and the wants of a woman, whereas homosexuals do not have that problem. However, I found in my psychology practice that gay partners can be every bit as jealous and possessive as straight partners. Perhaps that's why the number of gay couples choosing monogamy appears to have been increasing in the last 20 years. Cynics have claimed that this is merely a response to the reality of AIDS; I think it's more likely a byproduct of gays' increased integration into the larger society.

DRAG QUEENS AND FEMALE IMPERSONATORS

A small subgroup of homosexuals are the drag queens, gay men who like to dress up in varying parodies of female sexuality, and the female impersonators, whose aim is to create a perfect illusion of being a famous female. Many people became familiar with female impersonators by seeing Craig Russell, the female impersonator who starred in the hugely successful film *Outrageous*. Russell reproduced the appearance, physical movements, spoken and singing voices of famous females with almost uncanny accuracy. Except for his size, he actually seemed temporarily to become the women he imitated.

In the past, gay men have frequently felt uncomfortable, even hostile, about drag queens, probably because they feared that drag queens would convey the impression that gay men are either bogus women or confused men, objects fit for derision and ridicule. This fear seems to have lessened in recent years, as sexual minorities of all kinds have become more known and accepted. A current well-known and highly respected drag queen is the American RuPaul, popular singer and movie actor (and now also the spokesperson for MAC cosmetics, along with k. d. lang.)

DO FAMILIES "CAUSE" HOMOSEXUALITY?

Are certain families more likely to produce homosexual offspring? Three important studies — the San Francisco Bay area one by Bell and Weinberg, plus U.S. and British studies by Marvin Siegelman at City College of New York — tried to answer this question by examining the family backgrounds of straight and gay adults. The researchers could not find any common feature of the American or British family or of the person's upbringing that could have "caused" sexual orientation. They reported that most homosexuals in their studies were reared as heterosexuals in ordinary families that didn't appear to be different from the families that produced heterosexuals. Siegelman pointed out that studies in the 1960s and earlier, which described the mothers of homosexuals as "especially intimate, close binding and dominant" and the fathers as "detached, retiring, weak and rejecting," had recruited their subjects from mental health settings where the families were neurotic. Siegelman found that *only* with neurotic homosexuals were the parents more rejecting and less loving. The parents of psychologically normal homosexuals did not differ from the parents of heterosexuals.

I found the same thing in the gay men and women who were my patients. As far as I could tell, their family backgrounds were indistinguishable from the families of my straight patients. In my own family, two older sons are gay but the younger one, who's adopted, is straight. Our straight son has different genes from our other sons, but I don't think his family environment was significantly different from theirs.

Bell and Weinberg examined a number of popular notions about the cause of homosexuality and refuted them all. These notions included pressure from peers, being labelled as a sissy at an early age, having an unresolved Oedipus complex (thank you, Dr. Freud), having a father who was cold and detached, being seduced by an older person or having had bad experiences with the opposite sex. None of these factors appeared to have any influence on the development of a homosexual orientation. The authors noted that homosexual orientation often reveals itself in atypical childhoods (shy, unathletic boys and tomboyish girls). It is firmly established by the end of adolescence and resistant to change from outside influences.

In some studies both homosexual men and women have reported that their fathers had been cold and detached, but it's quite possible that the father's behaviour was a reaction to, rather than a cause of, the child's atypical interests and behaviour. Even if a father *is* cold and detached, there's no evidence that that would cause homosexuality. In a 1984 study by psychology professors Paul VanWyk and Chrisann Geist, the absence of either a father or a mother from a family accounted for less than one percent of the variance in adult sexual preference.

American psychiatrist Richard Isay, who has written extensively about his experience of doing psychotherapy with gay men, found nothing specific about the families of gay men that he did not also find in the families of straight men. Homosexual patients sometimes reported having families like those described in the psychoanalytic literature as being the cause of homosexuality — a strong, binding mother and/or a father perceived as being weak — but Isay found the same kinds of families in his heterosexual patients. What he did find that was unique to his homosexual patients was that every one of them reported having felt "different" from other children, from the age of three or four. The feeling was described as being "more sensitive, crying more easily, having his feelings hurt more readily, having more aesthetic interests and being less aggressive than others of his age." These feelings made them feel different from other children and sometimes different from their families as well.

My own two gay sons fit Isay's childhood profile in several respects. They were tender-hearted boys who shunned boyhood fights and team sports. Marc loved books and music: he played the piano well from an early age and devoured books as though they were cookies. His preference for books over rough-housing sometimes made it difficult for him to find childhood companions, but in high school he finally found a group like himself who preferred literature to linebacking. Christopher as a boy preferred drawing and painting to team sports, but most of all he loved animals, a large number and variety of which paraded through our lives over the years. Though Chris had boy playmates, he also had girls as friends, at an age when most other boys didn't. He sometimes got teased about that, but neither he nor we thought it was weird. In fact, I remember being pleased that my boys didn't dislike girls as most other boys did. I assumed we were raising non-sexist sons; it never occurred to me they might be gay.

Do families with pro-gay attitudes foster homosexuality in their offspring? A study by psychologists at Northwestern University suggests that even this kind of family doesn't promote homosexuality. Most pairs of gay brothers in this study reported that they had both been either feminine or masculine in childhood but, as adults, one of the pair might still be feminine while the other no longer was, or the other way round. This indicated that, whatever the family's influence on masculine or feminine behaviour, it was limited to childhood.

The study also found no support for the notion that having a gay brother can cause a boy to become homosexual. Participants reported being aware of their first homosexual feelings at age 11, on average, and had their first sexual involvement with a male at age 17, whereas they did not learn about their brother's homosexuality, on average, until age 21. The gay brothers did not report more distant relationships with their parents than reported by a comparison group. However, when compared to gay men who had no brothers, gay men with gay brothers expressed less self-acceptance of their homosexuality. (Given the prejudice against gay people, it's easy to imagine they felt unhappy about "burdening" their parents with more than one gay son. My own second gay son said exactly that when he finally came out as a gay man.)

What about children who are raised by gay or lesbian parents? Do these children have a greater chance of becoming homosexual adults? Apparently not. So far studies have focused on boys and have found that boys raised in households where the male parents were openly gay grew into heterosexual adults. The same was true for boys raised in openly lesbian households; there was no indication of sexual identity confusion in these boys, or of homosexual interest. The relationships these boys enjoyed with adult males were similar to the relationships enjoyed by boys raised in heterosexual households. The vast majority of children of lesbian and gay parents, like the majority of children of straight parents, are heterosexual. At the same time, most lesbians and gays have heterosexual parents. It's obvious that, whether parents are gay or straight, their sexual orientation cannot predict the sexual orientation of their children.

GAY AND LESBIAN PARENTS

Alison Brewin and Vanessa Jacobsen are a bright, hospitable lesbian couple in their mid-30s, who agreed to be interviewed for this book. They have two small children. The women have been together 10 years now — a comfortable couple who, in conversation, often fill in the blanks for one another. Even their looks appear complementary: Alison has dark curly hair, dark eyes and a pleasant roundness, while Vanessa has pale blue eyes and straight fair hair and a more athletic build. She is, in fact, a very accomplished golfer.

The two share child care. Alison, a former lawyer, currently works three days a week for West Coast LEAF (Legal Education and

Action Fund), a feminist organization that has established several important legal precedents for Canadian women in the past two decades. Vanessa, a commerce graduate, also works three days a week operating a toy store (It's All Fun and Games) jointly owned by herself and Alison. It's the only toy store on "The Drive," meaning Commercial Drive, the busy street running through the centre of the popular multi-ethnic area in old East Vancouver where Vanessa and Alison share a small comfortable house with Anders, their four-year-old son, and Molly, their one-year-old daughter. As we sat in their cozy living room, Anders and Molly trotted in and out, chased, giggled, showed toys, wrestled with Maggie, the black Labrador dog, and climbed up on laps for a cuddle. Alison is the one they call "Mom," while Vanessa is "Nessa." Watching the women with their children, it was easy to see the strong, close bond among them.

Alison says that, growing up, she had always looked forward to having a family someday, but once she realized she was a lesbian (at age 19), she thought children were no longer an option for her. But as the years went by, she gradually began to see that being a lesbian should not preclude her becoming a mother. She determined to make it happen, even if she had to go it alone. After she met Vanessa, however, she was prepared to wait until Vanessa, a few years younger than she, was also ready to become a parent. "I'd seen how great Vanessa was with our nieces and nephews and with the little kids who come into the toy store," recalls Alison. "I knew she'd be a good parent." After many months of discussion and a great deal of soul-searching, the couple agreed to take the plunge into parenthood.

But which of them would be the birth mother? More discussions. As Alison was eager to experience pregnancy, they decided that, for the first child at least, she would be the birth mother. That decision was harder for the second child, but again Alison was more enthusiastic about it than Vanessa, so ultimately they agreed that Alison would once again be the one to become pregnant. Vanessa says she has felt "intensely involved" in both of Alison's pregnancies and she hasn't ruled out the possibility of becoming pregnant herself if they were to want a third child sometime. "My mother and grandmother would be delighted," says Vanessa, "but I guess that's not really a good enough reason, so we'll see what happens in the future."

Having made the decision to become parents, the two women were faced with the challenge of finding a suitable father. Vanessa, whose own father was uninvolved in her life, would have been happy with a sperm donor. But Alison, who has a close relationship with her father, leaned toward the possibility of choosing a man who was known to them — someone they liked, a man who'd enjoy having some involvement with the children while respecting Alison and Vanessa as the two "hands-on" parents in charge.

The solution presented itself in the form of Grant Hurrle, a gay friend who was already part of their lives and seemed to be perfect for the role of biological father to their children. Alison describes Grant as "intelligent, kind, fun, decent — a lovely guy." "Besides," chimes in Vanessa, "he plays golf!" In fact, she and Grant were on the fairway the day Vanessa asked if he would be willing to play the special part Vanessa and Alison had in mind for him. Grant was delighted. He had always envied his brother for having children, assuming that he'd never have the same opportunity because he was gay. The proposal from Alison and Vanessa suited him perfectly. He happily accepted the rules they outlined: biological father, faithfully involved with the children but careful not to usurp the authority of their two female parents.

"We both felt some anxiety about the situation before the provincial government passed legislation permitting a same-sex parent to adopt," says Alison, "because you hear so many horror stories about lesbians losing their children. But when Vanessa was able to adopt the children, Grant gave up all his legal rights, and it's worked out really well. Thankfully, none of us is into staking out territory regarding the kids." The children carry their mothers' names — "Brewin

Jacobsen" — though their birth certificates list Alison and Grant as the biological parents.

Alison is quick to point out that she and Grant did not have sex in order for her to become pregnant. "We used the 'turkey baster' method," she says, referring to the plastic syringe that she and Vanessa filled with Grant's sperm that he had provided in a small jar.

The children call Grant "Dad" and delight in his company. He takes them at least once a week and often babysits to give Alison and Vanessa a night out. A travel agent, last year Grant took Anders to Eastern Canada to meet his parents — Anders' paternal grandparents — who live in a small rural town where gay people tend to be invisible. Grant says initially his parents had trouble "making sense of the arrangement," whereas Vanessa's and Alison's families, both of whom are urban, were more familiar with gay people and able to be more supportive of the arrangement from the beginning.

Reaction from other people has also been positive. "We've been really lucky," says Alison, "we have actually never had a negative comment." Strangers, referred by friends and relatives, sometimes call them at home for information about lesbian parenting. On several occasions, women from all over the province who have heard about Alison and Vanessa have come into their toy store, shyly seeking advice from Vanessa, both about being gay and about being a lesbian parent.

How will their children explain having two moms? I asked. "Well, so far we only have Anders' playschool experience to go by," says Alison. "One little boy said to him, 'I hear you have two mummies; maybe you'll have a hundred mummies!' Anders thought that was pretty funny." Vanessa adds, "Anders knows he has two moms; if we're out shopping and people refer to me as his mom, he's fine with that. As the kids get older, we'll just keep talking about it, telling them why Daddy doesn't live in our house, explaining that some families have a mom and a dad and other families have two moms or two dads or only one parent, and all of it's perfectly okay so long as they love each other." To which Alison adds, "What's a 'normal' family nowadays anyhow? The number of traditional families — mom and dad and kids living together — is declining rapidly in North America and there's getting to be a lot of different kinds of families, so I think our situation won't seem unusual in the future."

Stanley Alexander and Byron Chiefmoon are another homosexual couple raising children in Vancouver. Both men are in their 40s. They've been together for thirteen years. Byron — a tall, handsome Native man with black hair and dark eyes — grew up on a reserve in Alberta. He speaks in a quiet, measured way, often pausing to reflect before he responds to a question or comment. Stan is a pleasant, sandy-haired white man who grew up in an urban setting. Outgoing and extremely verbal, Stan is an interesting contrast to his partner. Yet despite their very different backgrounds, looks and personalities, the two men obviously have a strong, loving relationship. In conversation with them, I was impressed by their mutual admiration and respect, and by the pride they share in their children — two daughters, Daffney, 16, and Agatha, 12, and a 14-year-old son, Davy.

Byron and Stan became parents 10 years ago, when they assumed the "temporary" care of Byron's sister's children. Separated from her husband, the children's mother was trying to get her life "back on track." Byron welcomed the chance to bring children into the home; he'd grown up in a family of nine and had always hoped to have a family himself. Stan wasn't so sure at first, but when he met baby Agatha, the first of the three to join them, it was "love at first sight." "I discovered what it means to love unconditionally and to have that love returned by a child," says Stan. "It's wonderful."

After two years, it became apparent that the children were here to stay: the mother had moved on to other things and, with her consent, Byron became the children's permanent legal guardian and Stan their de facto dad. For Stan, becoming a parent was an unexpected blessing: "My family always accepted my gayness," he says, "but they never expected I'd have kids and neither did I, so this was a bonus for them and of course for me. My mom considers our kids to be her grandchildren."

Previously the family lived on Vancouver Island, where Byron and Stan owned and operated a coffee-roasting business and coffee shop. After Stan was involved in a serious automobile accident, they were forced to sell the business and move to Vancouver. Stan enrolled at Simon Fraser University and is now studying for a degree in communications. Seeing how much Stan was enjoying his studies, Byron decided to go back to school, too, first studying film at Capilano College and now dance and film at Simon Fraser University.

I asked the children whether they called both of the men Dad. "No, we just call them by their names," said Agatha, "but I did call Byron 'Mom' for a few years. I was only two years old when I came to live with him and Stan, and Byron did all the mom things — the cooking and grocery shopping and sewing our clothes and all that — so I just thought he was a mom." These household chores were not new to Byron; he had always been more interested in women's work than he was in men's work: "I knew from an early age that I was different," he says now. "I was a boy who liked dolls and cooking and disliked the rough kinds of things other boys did." He grew up to be a talented actor and dancer, and eventually founded his own dance company.

The children have obviously benefited from Byron's artistic interests. Davy plays the trumpet, Daffney the violin, and Agatha studies singing and takes part in school musical productions. One summer they all spent a month at the Banff School of Fine Arts in the Canadian Rockies, where Byron's dance company was in residence.

Like many other couples, straight and gay, the two men divide the household chores along traditional lines. Byron is the cook, grocery shopper, disciplinarian, buyer of kids' clothes and supervisor of

their chores. Stan looks after the garden, the dog, the house mainte-
nance and the garbage. "I can cook, too, if I have to," says Stan, "and
I do when Byron's away with his dance company, but I'm just not as
organized about that kind of stuff as Byron is."

What's it like having two dads? I asked the children. They
seemed puzzled by the question. Then Daffney said, "At our school
there's all different kinds of families. Lots of them don't have a dad
and a mom, so we're not really different." Davy loyally added, "We're
proud of them."

Do you ever get teased about having gay parents? I asked the children. Both girls said no, they'd never heard a word of criticism. Davy
said, "Once a guy at school said something to me, but it doesn't matter." Later, when I asked Byron and Stan about the incident, they
told me that a schoolmate had said to Davy, "You've got two dads, so
they must be fags. And that means you're a fag, too!" Davy reported
the incident to the teacher and after school told Stan how angry he
was to hear him and Byron called fags. Surprised, Stan asked, "But
Davy, you do know that Byron and I are gay, don't you?" And Davy
said, "Yes, sure, but that doesn't mean you're *fags*!" Clearly, in Davy's
mind, being gay was no ground for insult.

One thing that struck me about this gay-parents family was its
similarity to most of the straight families I've known: two parents, several children, regular bedtimes, pets, music lessons, chores and
weekly allowances. This family also has a biweekly family meeting
where anyone can raise issues for discussion. "It's a respectful time,"
says Stan, "a time where we review how we're treating one another."

During the 10 years they've been parents, Byron and Stan have
lived in a rural setting, a suburban setting and (now) in a big city.
They told me that, in none of those settings, have they ever had trouble because of their unconventional family. "The schools have
always been completely supportive," Stan told me, "and so have our
neighbours. I've learned from this experience that the vast majority

of people — in Canada at least — are not homophobic. If you're friendly to them, they'll be friendly to you."

Are kids raised by gay or lesbian parents really psychologically okay? To answer this question, psychologist Bonnie Strickland at the University of Massachusetts at Amherst reviewed a number of studies of gay and lesbian families. She found that the overall emotional well-being of homosexuals and their children was as psychologically healthy as that of their heterosexual counterparts. Another report, this one out of Widener University at Wilmington, Delaware, compared 15 lesbian couples and the three- to nine-year-old children born to them through donor insemination, with 15 matched heterosexual couples and their children of similar ages. A variety of tests were used to evaluate the children's cognitive functioning and behaviour; no significant differences were found between the two groups. Researchers also found no difference in the quality of the marital relationship between lesbian and heterosexual couples, but the lesbian couples exhibited more "parenting awareness" skills than the heterosexual couples.

Other research comparing children raised by homosexual parents to those raised by heterosexual parents has found no differences in the children's sexual identity as male or female, their gender role development as "typical" men or women, their social relationships or their mental health.

Judging from the results of such studies, it looks as though family rearing has little or no effect on what sexual orientation a child will have when grown to adulthood. What does seem to be a predisposing factor to homosexuality is childhood gender nonconformity (behaving like the opposite sex), which apparently occurs regardless of the kind of family the child is born into. Psychiatrist Richard Green at the University of California followed 66 effeminate boys and 56 masculine boys for 15 years, to see how they would turn out. Despite the fact that most of the parents of the "sissy" boys tried to discourage their sons' effeminate behaviour, and some of the parents even obtained treatment for their sons, 66 percent of the boys seen at follow-up had turned out to be homosexual, transsexual or transvestite, whereas only one of the masculine boys was homosexual. As for the boys who received psychological treatment, about three-quarters of them as adults were gay or transsexual; in fact, a slightly *greater* proportion of those who received treatment turned out to be non-heterosexual than the boys who received no treatment at all. (That doesn't mean, of course, that treatment *caused* their sexual orientation. It's more likely that parents of those children with more extremely atypical behaviour would seek treatment.)

Several other studies have also reported a strong link between childhood gender nonconformity and homosexuality in adulthood, especially for males. But these studies also found that some gay men as children were just as gender-typical as other children; it's been proposed that homosexuality may be less biological for them. Lesbians report moderately more childhood tomboyism than other women do, but a large number of straight women also recall a tomboy childhood. In gay adults, too, there are marked individual differences in their overall masculinity and femininity, as well as individual differences among various psychological characteristics. A person may be feminine in some characteristics but typically masculine or even super-masculine in others.

WHAT KEEPS HOMOSEXUALITY IN THE HUMAN GENE POOL?

This is an intriguing question for biologists. Why would homosexuality persist in the human gene pool when homosexuals are much less likely to produce offspring? Biologists usually measure "fitness" in terms of an individual's likelihood of reproducing and passing along his genes. Since homosexuals don't generally reproduce, their biological "fitness" quotient should be quite low. Why then hasn't the incidence of homosexuality gradually diminished and eventually disappeared?

Some social scientists believe that homosexuality continues in the gene pool because it's the product of social forces. But if that's the case, why hasn't homosexuality dramatically increased, now that most Western cultures are more tolerant of it than they formerly were? Instead, the prevalence of homosexuality has apparently remained pretty constant, at least in the U.S., where most of the studies have been done.

Several writers have speculated about male homosexuality's survival in the gene pool (so far there's virtually no such speculation about lesbianism). It's been suggested there was probably survival value for the earliest human males in having some of their number who were less aggressive and more sensitive and communicative. (If all of those males had been aggressive, the race might not have survived!) A more recent version of this idea by Edward Miller at the University of New Orleans argues that a strong dose of certain prenatal female hormones could shift a male fetus in the direction of homosexuality. A weaker dose, however, could produce a heterosexual male who's more sensitive, kind and empathic. Miller says that's just the kind of man women would choose to have children with, so the "feminine" genes of that kind of man would be passed along to the next generation, where offspring would have an increased likelihood of being gay.

Some academics have speculated that gay genes persist because they confer some benefit — perhaps creativity, for example — on our species. It's common knowledge that there are many more gay men in all of the creative arts than their relatively small numbers would warrant. Others argue that genes for homosexuality endure because variety is crucial to all species. The more diverse we are, the more likely it is that some of us will be able to adapt to a changing environment. (This is the "biological exuberance" of which Bruce Bagemihl writes.)

All of these theories are just that at the moment — theories. It remains to be seen whether any of them will lead to empirical studies.

LESBIANS

Unfortunately, much less is known about lesbians than about gay men because lesbians have been much less studied. One thing that's apparent from surveys is that there are fewer lesbians than gay men — perhaps even half or two-thirds as many. So far there's no definitive explanation for this discrepancy, though it's been noted that males outnumber females in a wide variety of anomalies (see Chapter 6).

Several studies have suggested that lesbianism has a biological basis. For one thing, lesbians in the Kinsey study were, on average, taller and heavier than heterosexual women, although there was no difference in the age of puberty. More recently, British researchers working out of a fertility clinic in London reported that almost 80 percent of the lesbians who came for treatment had polycystic ovaries (polycystic ovarian syndrome), compared to only 32 percent of the heterosexual patients. One of the main features of this female condition is an abnormally high level of male sex hormones, which can give women excess body hair, a deeper voice and less breast tissue. The researchers hypothesized that the excessively high male hormone might have been a predisposing factor for lesbianism in these women.

Another difference in lesbians is that they have significantly less right-handedness than straight women. When Kenneth Zucker in the Department of Psychiatry at the University of Toronto combined the results of 20 previous handedness studies, he found that lesbians were nearly twice as likely as straight women to be non-right-handed. As hand preference originates in the womb, these results suggest that lesbian orientation, at least in some women, has early neurobiological roots.

Also pointing to a biological basis is the fact that lesbians have more homosexual relatives than other women. On the other hand, most brain functions in lesbians are organized like those of other women, whereas in gay men several of these functions are organized like those of females.

Women tend to come to lesbianism later in life than men come to homosexuality. Perhaps adolescent lesbians, being female, tend to interpret their feelings for other girls as friendship rather than erotic love. On average, girls did not suspect they were lesbian until they were 18, and didn't define themselves as lesbian until their early 20s.

Some lesbians have no memories of early same-sex attractions and report that such attractions were triggered in adulthood by exposure to same-sex individuals or ideas, or by experiencing a very intense emotional attachment to a particular woman. Among lesbians who do recall early same-sex attractions, most studies have found that the earliest attractions occurred when they were about 10 or 12, the same age heterosexual children first experience sexual feelings. (These early feelings coincide with maturation of the adrenal glands.)

Compared to gay men, higher percentages of lesbians have had heterosexual sex. It's been reported that four-fifths of gay women, compared to only about half of gay men, have had heterosexual intercourse (typically because of social pressure from family and friends) before abandoning the heterosexual life and coming out as homosexual. Also, a higher percentage of lesbians marry before eventually declaring their homosexuality. In the Bell and Weinberg study described earlier, only half of the lesbian women rated their feelings and attractions as exclusively gay. The researchers estimated that more than a third of the lesbians they studied were involved in some current heterosexual activity which they found pleasurable, despite having a predominantly lesbian lifestyle. Psychiatrist Richard Pillard found that the women aged 25 to 40 whom he studied were reluctant to label themselves as homosexual or heterosexual, which was not true of the men in the study. "The women's sexual feelings seemed to depend more upon the partner they were with," Pillard later commented. "... [I]n general, they seemed to have the ability for a 'situational response,' which the men lacked."

In the decade following this study, several other researchers observed the same phenomenon. Psychologist Lisa Diamond and anthropologist Ritch Savin-Williams reported that two-thirds of the lesbian women they studied had experienced periodic attractions to men. In other women they studied, who did not call themselves lesbian, one of the most common triggers for same-sex involvement was an intense, emotionally intimate relationship — for example, one participant became sexually involved with her best friend. "We've known each other since we were 12 and we've always been really affectionate, but last Tuesday it just sort of kept going ... Right now I only have these feelings for her, and I don't know if that'll change. I don't know if I'm a lesbian. I just know I want to be with her, forever." The researchers noted that, two years later, this woman and her best friend had resumed being platonic friends; they identified as heterosexual and never experienced attractions for other women. Another woman in this study reported that "her 'gut level' attractions for men were stronger than her attractions for women, [but] she consistently achieved greater levels of emotional intimacy with women than men. Because this was important to her, she eventually identified as lesbian."

As noted earlier, many women who call themselves lesbians describe their sexuality as a personal choice. More than half of the sample of lesbians in one study (Rosenbluth, 1997) perceived their homosexuality as resulting from a conscious, deliberate choice. Other studies have reported similar findings. Moreover, when women's physiological responses to scenes of both heterosexual sex and lesbian sex were measured, there was no difference between the response of lesbians and of heterosexual women; both groups of women responded more strongly to scenes of heterosexual sex than lesbian sex. These findings seems to suggest that, for many women, identifying as a lesbian may have less to do with erotic attraction than with other factors. Claudette Charbonneau and Patricia Lander reported that a third of the women in their sample who converted to lesbianism during midlife cited "reading feminist texts" as a reason for doing so. Perhaps not surprisingly, those women who *chose* lesbianism had a more difficult adjustment than those who became lesbian through self-discovery.

Writer Marcia Kaye described a 49-year-old woman named Sheila who, after 15 years of marriage, followed by "long periods of celibacy, punctuated by two torrid affairs," met Carmen, an attractive gay hairstylist her age with whom she fell in love and had now been living for seven years. "I still have the greatest admiration for men," said Sheila, "but I fell in love with a person who just happens to be a woman." Other women described by Kaye made comments such as, "Her gender was almost immaterial." Researchers who studied these women reported that the loving relationship was much more important to them than the sex.

It seems obvious from the above studies that lesbians are much more of a "mixed bag" than gay men. While some studies point to a biological basis for lesbianism in some women, other studies suggest that different factors are the determinants for other women. (This is an important distinction from gay men, the majority of whom report that they had no choice in their sexual orientation.) In the decades following the 1960s and the feminist revolution, some women chose lesbianism to oppose male patriarchy and join with other women in the struggle for female equality. Since then many women have chosen lesbianism for personal reasons that have little or nothing to do with either feminist politics or biology. Some of these women identify themselves as lesbians and live a lesbian lifestyle, but erotic attraction is low or non-existent in their list of reasons for doing so. What's needed in future research is a separation of the subtypes of lesbianism for study, instead of trying to draw conclusions about lesbians in general from assorted samples of them.

In terms of sexual techniques, lesbian couples may be less adventurous than others. Lesbians have reported that they prefer hugging, kissing, cuddling and other nongenital kinds of sexual expression to genital sex. In one study, 61 percent of lesbian couples reported they had oral sex infrequently or not at all. Most couples in the study limited themselves to manual stimulation and tribadism (rubbing one's genitals against the other person's body).

Overall, lesbians do not appear to have pervasive sexual problems but they do report notably low frequency of sex. Psychotherapist and author JoAnn Loulan of San Francisco surveyed almost 1,600 lesbians and found that 25 percent had been celibate for one to five years, and eight percent for six years or more. Sociologists Philip Blumstein and Pepper Schwartz found that lesbians in long-term committed relationships had sex far less frequently than any other type of couple studied. Only about a third of those in relationships of two years or more had sex at least once a week, and 47 percent of those in relationships of more than five years had sex only once a month or less. Perhaps this is not surprising, considering that many women who call themselves lesbians are motivated by factors other than erotic attraction to women.

· Some investigators have suggested that the low frequency of sex among lesbians may simply be due to the fact that they are women. Perhaps the frequencies of sex viewed as normal in long-term heterosexual couples are largely the result of males initiating sex and females acquiescing. Sexologists report that women in general appear to be less interested in sex than men, and all surveys of sexual behaviour show that women, overall, are less sexually active than men. It's been suggested that the apparent discrepancy in sexual interest between women and men may actually reflect different prefences — a male preference for orgasmic genital sex and a female preference for nongenital kinds of sexual expression.

Ruth Fassinger at the University of Maryland and Susan Morrow at Columbia University summarized the research findings from the 1980s and 1990s about lesbian relationships: lesbian couples are generally flexible in the roles they play and prefer relationships in which power is equally shared; they often experience a general lack of social support, especially from their families; they are more likely to be satisfied with their relationship if both partners are "out" regarding their lesbianism. Although they report having problems maintaining individual autonomy in a relationship, they also report high levels of relationship satisfaction, trust and commitment.

For most lesbians, sex has tended to be closely bound to love, as it has for heterosexual women. The choice of a partner, therefore, has usually focused on affection and emotional closeness rather than on physical attributes and age. This is quite different from the partner choices of men. Both gay and straight men tend to put a high premium on physical attractiveness and a youthful appearance.

Before the late 19th century, the term "lesbian" was largely unknown, although "romantic friendships" were common between single upper-middle-class women in the 18th and 19th centuries (described in Lillian Faderman's fascinating book, *Surpassing the Love of Men*). These women did not regard themselves as lesbians but they frequently shared lifelong companionships with other women — called "Boston marriages" after author Henry James wrote about them in *The Bostonians*. Faderman concludes that these relationships were emotionally passionate and more intimate than heterosexual marriages, but they generally did not involve sex. Besides providing companionship, these relationships often enabled the women in them to have some kind of intellectual or career interest which would not have been possible in the traditional heterosexual marriage of their day.

Around the turn of the 20th century in America, a number of "passing women" (as they were called) emerged. These women (described by Jonathan Katz in *Gay American History*) dressed as men and took male names for themselves. Some of them even took on male identities throughout their lives, "married" other women and passed as men until their true sex was revealed at death. Whether they were lesbians, transsexuals or neither is not known.

In the 1950s, lesbians often assumed rigid "butch-femme" roles in their relationships. It's been suggested these roles were simply imitations of heterosexual couples and would pass once lesbians became more comfortable and more public with their relationships. For most lesbians that's just what happened, but even today in some lesbian relationships there are "femmes" who occupy the female role and "butches" who assume the male role. Butches usually dress in men's clothing and often have male nicknames such as Lou, Sid or Billy. The book *Dagger on Butch Women*, by Lily Burana and Roxxie and Linnea Due, includes interviews with butch lesbians. One says, "I always knew that I was going to fall in love with a woman and get married and be the husband ... I knew I was a girl but not like other girls." Another describes competing and fighting with other butches for the same woman. "We had to make a rule that whoever saw a girl first had first rights." Another describes having felt ashamed of her breasts until she discovered that her femme lover admired them. I suspect (as others have suggested) that some butches may not be lesbians at all, but transsexuals — female bodies with male identities.

In the past 25 years, lesbian radicals, like their radical heterosexual counterparts, have consciously emphasized the separation of sex and love, which they see as traditional female sex conditioning. Other "outlyers" in the lesbian community — the drag kings (women dressing up as men), the stone butches, the dyke leather daddies — boldly and proudly define themselves as "queers" and are often disdainful of lesbians and gays who have sought to downplay their gay identity and become assimilated into the mainstream.

In recent years the phenomenon of drag kings has entered the entertainment world in bars and concert stages. Most drag kings are lesbian or bisexual women, but some straight women are also beginning to show up in the drag king scene, just as they're showing up in the bisexual scene. These women have not altered their heterosexual orientation; they're simply having fun imitating the opposite sex, in the same way as straight men have done for years.

FOUR SEXES INSTEAD OF TWO?

Some writers have argued that butch lesbians and effeminate gay men are actually two additional sexes and we should add these two to "male" and "female" to describe the true array of human sexuality. While I like the idea of getting beyond penis-equals-masculine and vagina-equals-feminine, I'd argue against expanding from two sexes to four because four would still be far too few to describe all of the variants in human sexuality. What about the bisexuals, the trans-sexuals and the intersexuals described in the next chapter? How about the subcategories of heterosexuals who haven't been studied yet, including straight men who are super-feminine and straight women who are super-masculine?

Rather than merely adding on a couple of new categories to our existing classification system, I believe what we need is a paradigm shift to start us thinking in terms of an *array* of sexualities, some obvious and some subtle. As Anne Fausto-Sterling, Professor of Biology and Women's Studies at Brown University, writes: "... masculine and feminine cannot be parsed as some kind of continuum. Rather, sex and gender are best conceptualized as *points in a multidimensional space.*" (Emphasis added.)

4

Multiple Sexualities—
The Minors

Every divergence deserves to be cherished, simply
because it widens the bounds of life.
KAREL CAPEK, *Letters from Spain*

ISEXUALS, TRANSSEXUALS, INTERSEXUALS —
these are the three best-known players in the
minor sex league. "Minor" here refers to
numbers, of course, not to importance. Perhaps I should use the
term "rare" instead of "minor" for people in these groups. Of the
three, bisexuals are the least rare.

Bisexuals

These are people whose genitals and self-identity are the same sex,
and who are erotically attracted to *both* sexes, to about the same
degree. It's hard to say how many people fit into this category, but the
number is probably quite small. More people may describe themselves as bisexual and have sexual relations with both sexes, but they

usually have strong physiological arousal to only one sex or the other. This is especially true of men. Kurt Freund, the plethysmograph man whose work was described in Chapter 3, said that his many investigations over more than 25 years led him to conclude that, though some people may engage in sexual activity with both sexes, very few actually show erotic physical responses to both. He emphasized the importance of distinguishing between what arouses individuals and what they *do*. In his own research (men only) he did not find any men who were about equally aroused by pictures of naked men and pictures of naked women.

Some gay men and women have had extensive heterosexual experience due to social expectations and pressure from family and friends, but that doesn't mean they're bisexual. In retrospect these people will report that they always had stronger erotic feelings for their own sex but resisted acting upon them, hoping they could be straight. Sometimes such people have played the role of heterosexual person for many years before they were finally able to accept their gay identity.

Same-sex experiences also often occur in the course of adolescent experimentation, especially in boys, but the young people involved don't identify themselves as anything but heterosexual. At other times same-sex behaviour is situational — for example, in prisons or the army, as noted in Chapter 2 — but in the large majority of such incidents people do not experience enduring erotic attraction to both sexes, nor do they identify themselves as bisexual.

Bisexuality used to be largely ignored or scoffed at. Lesbians and gay men often accused self-proclaimed bisexuals of trying to hang onto heterosexual privilege by avoiding admitting they were homosexual. Since the late 1980s, however, bisexuals have asserted their separate identity more publicly and there is now much greater recognition and acceptance of bisexuality, either as a separate orientation or as a universal human option.

Unfortunately, bisexuals have not been extensively studied. Most of the earlier studies of sexual orientation simply lumped bisexuals in with homosexuals and anybody else who wasn't heterosexual. Clearly, this is not a useful method for learning about any group. (Reminds me of my days in graduate school, when I was advised by one professor not to include women in my research because they "mess up the data," meaning that they obtain different scores from men.)

In the studies that have looked at bisexuals separately from other groups, all have observed that bisexuals are often different from both heterosexuals and homosexuals. On personality tests, bisexual women score in a more masculine and less feminine direction than both lesbian and straight women. This has been attributed to abnormal exposure to male hormones in the womb, as several studies have found a high number of bisexuals among women who, for various reasons, had been so exposed. Remember the DES girls in Chapter 1, whose mothers had taken the synthetic hormone DES to prevent miscarriage? When these girls grew up, their behaviour was more masculine in various ways and more of them were homosexual than would be expected, and even more of them were bisexual.

The average bisexual woman tends to realize she's bisexual at a later time than the average lesbian realizes she's a lesbian. One study found that those lesbians who'd ever thought of themselves as bisexual gave up thinking so at the average age of 25. In contrast, the average bisexual woman in the study who had ever wondered if she was lesbian was almost 30 before she finally identified herself as bisexual.

There are all sorts of theories about bisexuality, but not much hard evidence. Biologist James Weinrich, who's also a certified sexologist, proposed in the 1980s that there are two kinds of sexual attraction: romantic love, which he called "limerant," and physical attraction, which he called "lust." He said the typical woman who calls herself bisexual can probably feel romantic love for either women or men. She may feel lust for only one of them or perhaps lust isn't all that important to her. The typical bisexual man probably feels lust only for men but can feel romantic love for women too.

Recently psychology professor Lisa Diamond extended Weinrich's theory. For his "romantic love and lust," she substitutes "love and desire." She claims the two are functionally independent — that is, a person can "fall in love" without experiencing sexual desire, and can experience sexual desire without falling in love. She also views "falling in love" as not being intrinsically oriented toward one sex or the other; in other words, either sex can fall in love with both sexes. Finally, she believes that both love and desire can lead to each other. Consequently, people can fall in love as a result of sexual desire (not too surprising), but they can also *develop* sexual desire as the result of falling in love. This is particularly true for women, says Diamond; she notes that women frequently say they fell in love with a *person* rather than with a man or a woman.

I think Weinrich and Diamond are right about two kinds of love, but I wouldn't define romantic love as "sexual." People may be swept into a sexual relationship by a powerful emotional bond to someone, but in my experience it's extremely difficult to sustain a sexual relationship based solely on that. The finding that long-term lesbian couples have less sex than any other kind of couple supports that.

Bisexuals tend to have male and female partners sequentially rather than being sexually involved with both at the same time. A bisexual may be in a sexual relationship with a man for a few years and then switch to a sexual relationship with a woman, or vice versa. Isabella's story, below, seems typical.

A BISEXUAL WOMAN'S STORY
(Names have been changed, by request.)

Isabella is a 34-year-old corporate trainer for an insurance firm. She's a small, slim, blond woman with a pretty face and a quick smile. Socially at ease, she slips off her shoes and sits cross-legged on the sofa opposite me while we talk. Obviously bright, she weighs each question carefully.

"Am I a bisexual?" she asks with a laugh. "I don't know. I've never really called myself anything, except when I was 'required' to label myself to suit my partner. I just think of myself as a person. How about if I just tell you about my experience and see what you think my label should be?"

Isabella describes her childhood as "pretty typical" — two loving parents, two older brothers plus her twin brother, all of whom got along well and who still enjoy one another's company. "I liked having girlfriends when I was growing up," says Isabella, "but I also liked playing basketball and other sports that my brothers played," she recalls. Her only "difference," she thinks, was that she always liked the new and the different, and was always pushing the limits. "I wanted to be accepted by other people," she says, "but I didn't want to follow the beaten path. I read different books, listened to different music, was more curious than other people." In her teens, although Isabella went along with societal expectations to date boys, she was always curious about the local gay bar.

But it was not until her second year of university that Isabella got to know a homosexual person. Among her close circle of women friends, one — Susan — surprised everyone by declaring herself a lesbian. "I remember thinking 'this is neat,' recalls Isabella, "It was different, unusual, new. I was proud to have a gay friend; I could hardly wait to tell my family and my other friends." Isabella started going to gay bars with Susan and found that she liked the people there. "They were fun, friendly, open about expressing themselves — I liked that." Even so, she continued to date boys all through university. "I thought about being with a woman and we talked about it a lot in my group, because of Susan. I used to say, 'I'd like to try it just for one night to see what it's like.' I enjoyed women's company more, I liked their opinions, I appreciated their concern and their interest in me as a person."

Meanwhile, she continued her earlier relationship with Wes, "a wonderful man" about whom she had confused feelings. One night, shortly after graduation from university, Isabella met a woman at one of Susan's parties to whom she was strongly attracted. "She was interesting," says Isabella, "more artistic and intellectual than Wes." They kissed that night, but the woman was reluctant to pursue the relationship, as Isabella was still unsure about her own sexual orientation. After a brief separation from Wes, she went back to him for another two years, until she was 24. "But I was always wondering what else was out there," Isabella says. After she went to work in the banking profession, she met a lot of attractive men and decided to break off the relationship with Wes. She began dating men "from 18 to 52," but she felt no sexual attraction for any of them "except one, but then when it happened it was icky."

Then, on a visit to Vancouver, where Susan had relocated, Isabella met Sabine. "It was total fireworks between us," she remembers. "I had my first real orgasm with Sabine. I thought I had finally found what I was looking for." Like the other lesbians to whom Isabella had felt attracted, Sabine was "boyish-looking, but still feminine."

Isabella defined herself as a "lipstick lesbian" when she was involved with Sabine, because it made Sabine feel good and also because she felt societal pressure to do so. "I've never really wanted to define myself as anything," she says now, "but I wanted to be open that I too was in a committed relationship, just like the rest of the world."

The relationship lasted six years, then ended for a number of reasons: "Although Sabine and I loved each other dearly," Isabella says, "we weren't right for one another. Also, there was very little sex. Almost all the lesbians I knew who were in long-term relationships had experienced the same thing, but that didn't make it any easier to accept."

After breaking with Sabine, Isabella dated a few women, but nothing serious. "I noticed that the sexual attraction for women wasn't instant," she says. "It grew out of friendship and emotional attachment, whereas with men the sexual attraction came first and then — maybe — the other things."

Eventually Isabella started dating men again. Through some mutual friends she met Lee, her current love interest. "For the first time I feel I've connected on several levels," she says. "Physically, emotionally, spiritually and intellectually. We share the same values. He's communicative in the way women are communicative, but he's also a big manly man. I'm more mature now — I know what I like — and I like the person Lee is. He's a great person who just happens to be a man."

Before I can put the question, she does it for me. "Will I ever fall in love with a woman again? I don't know. I didn't fall in love with Lee the man, I fell in love with Lee the person. That's how it is with me."

When the interview ends, she slips into her fashionable jacket and rides off on her motorcycle.

ARE BISEXUALS MORE HIGHLY SEXED?

Looks as though they are. When researchers showed bisexuals pictures that normally arouse heterosexuals, they found that the bisexuals were more sexually aroused by these pictures than the straight people were. In other studies comparing bisexuals to gay and straight groups, the bisexuals reported higher rates of sexual activity and sexual fantasy, and greater levels of erotic interest, than both of the other groups. These results indicate that bisexuals are simply more interested in sex per se, which may have resulted from their having received unusual doses of sex hormones before birth.

BISEXUAL MEN VERSUS WOMEN

One of the most curious findings about bisexuality is that it's reported much more often by women than men. Men in most studies have generally identified as either straight or gay and only rarely as bisexual, whereas in some studies almost a third of the women have scored in the bisexual range on the Kinsey scale and other reporting tools. However, bisexuality was assessed in these studies on the basis of self-reported behaviour; there were no objective measures of bodily arousal to sexy pictures of men and women to determine whether these women actually were strongly attracted to both sexes. It is, of course, physically easier for women than men to have sex with both sexes: whereas men generally need to feel erotic attraction to perform sexually, women can be passive recipients engaging in sexual activity for reasons other than erotic attraction. In one study nearly all of the women over age 25 reported having engaged in sex when they had no desire for it.

The surprisingly large number of women who report bisexual feelings and behaviour has led some researchers to conclude that, for women, bisexuality is a stable orientation almost as common as heterosexuality. In other studies, however, the number of people, male or female, who identified as bisexual was very small. For example, in the big 1994 Chicago University survey described in the previous chapter, fewer than 1 percent of those surveyed identified themselves as bisexual.

I think the discrepancy in numbers is probably due to the way in which bisexuality is defined. Some people label themselves bisexual but in fact engage only in straight or gay sex. Calling themselves bisexual is a political statement about being inclusive. Women may think they're bisexual because they feel emotionally close to other women and either confuse these feelings with sexual attraction or decide that emotional closeness is more important than erotic attraction. Some homosexual men will sometimes have sex with women, but they remain primarily sexually attracted to other men. Among those men are, in my opinion, most of the married men in the past who called themselves bisexual but were actually gay men making a social accommodation to marriage, sometimes in order to have children.

BISEXUAL POLITICS

Bisexual politics today rejects the notion that sexual orientation is innate, and instead endorses "the fluidity of sexual orientation and gender" and "polyamory" (non-monagamy) for both sexes. At a bisexuality conference at the University of British Columbia in 2002, several speakers and workshops promoted this view. One workshop entitled "The Genderless Orgasm" advanced the belief that sex is intrinsically good and should be enjoyed with both sexes, at least until a person comes to identify "with whichever orientation fits best." That's also the view of Bert Archer, author of *The End of Gay*, who urges us to drop the sexual orientation labels from our collective psyche and endorse sex with both sexes. He writes, "In a society that has pretty successfully separated sex from reproduction and even, to a large extent, from its role as a stable basis of social propagation, the door's been left open for sex to be a lot more fun than it has been in millennia."

Harvard professor Marjorie Garber calls bisexuality the "default" orientation. She cites the experience of many writers, artists and performers — Frida Kahlo, Virginia Woolf, Oscar Wilde, W. H. Auden, Leonard Bernstein, Madonna — who have had sexual relationships with both women and men. She believes that bisexuality is about to be more widely accepted and practised in our society, as MTV and advertising promote ambiguous and fetishized images of men and women, encouraging today's young people to respond erotically to both sexes. "We are in a bisexual moment," says Garber, who defines bisexuality in terms of behaviour, not erotic orientation.

Certainly a growing number of young people today are playing with sexual variety and describing themselves as bisexual. Since the early 1990s it's become trendy for college students (especially women who participate in the club scene) to endorse "bisexual chic," sometimes based on the belief that many rock stars are bisexual. Some of these women claim a bisexual identity even without having sex with both men and women; others do have sex with both but only on a transitional, temporary basis. In a culture that promotes the notion of "getting everything you can," sex with both men and women may simply seem like a smarter option.

This book takes the position that bisexuality is not a universal potential. Just because people are willing to have sex with both males and females does not mean that they are erotically attracted to both, which I believe is the proper definition of bisexuality. However, I do realize there's a problem with refuting the claim of a universal bisexual potential. People's sexual orientation is not defined until late puberty or adulthood, after they've been exposed to years of socialization. It is possible that many more people are born with bisexual potential but are socialized into heterosexuality because that is the dominant cultural norm. At the present time, however, this is purely speculation.

Most studies of bisexuality so far have been descriptive and dependent upon self-reporting, which can sometimes be quite unreliable. There are signs, though, that more hard data may soon be available. Neuroscientists have found that mammals and birds have evolved three separate but related systems in the brain for lust, attraction and male-female attachment. These three systems underlie mating, reproduction and parenting. Now a group of researchers in New Jersey and New York have begun using MRIs of the human brain to identify the neural circuits associated with romantic attraction between people. Hopefully, in a few years, science will enable us to be much more definitive about the dynamics of bisexuality, and perhaps of other sexual orientations as well.

Transsexuals

In recent years there's been a tendency for sexual activists in academia, in the arts and in self-proclaimed "queer" communities to lump *all* non-heterosexual groups under the umbrella term "transgender," in a bid for greater inclusivity in the non-heterosexual community.

It's also become popular with some young people to engage in "gender-bending" or "fashionable androgyny" — deliberately toying with other people's perceptions of their sex by altering their style of dress, or by using makeup and other props. These are *social* phenomena, of course; they don't alter the intrinsic sexual identity of the people involved. These people are not transsexuals.

Transsexuals are men and women with typical male and female bodies but an inward identity that's at odds with the physical body. This isn't simply a matter of feeling more or less feminine or masculine. Transsexuals often report that, from their earliest childhood, they were convinced they were the wrong sex, "a woman trapped in a man's body" or vice versa. Some insisted on wearing the clothes of the opposite sex from a very early age, choosing games and other activities typical of the opposite sex, and resisting all parental attempts to make them dress and behave in accordance with their physical bodies.

As Blaine Beemer, a psychiatric nurse formerly with the Vancouver Hospital's Centre for Sexual Medicine, wrote:

An anatomically female transsexual … typically shuns frilly girl accoutrements for boys' wear; prefers GI Joe to Barbie; prefers playing baseball with the boys to baking with mom; and will only play house if she can be the dad, or the husband or brother. Many transsexuals actually assumed, in childhood, that they were the opposite sex, and that puberty magically would lead to the secondary sexual characteristics they so admired in the preferred gender. For the anatomical female, the onset of menstruation and breast growth comes as a huge disappointment and cruel confirmation of the biological truth.

Young transsexual men shun rough-and-tumble play, dress up in their mother's or sister's clothes, and may obsessively fantasize that they are a princess or mermaid. They gravitate to girls' games, such as skipping rope and playing house … they decide that it is more proper to sit rather than stand to urinate. They prefer the company of females, and become distraught when beard growth and a deeper voice destroy the fragile image they hold of themselves as a girl.

These children suffer from Gender Identity Disorder (GID), an intense desire to be the opposite sex. Often they also have a distinctive physical appearance that's different from other children. At the Clarke Institute of Psychiatry in Toronto, judges were asked to rate the physical appearance of boys and girls with and without GID. The raters didn't know which of the children had GID and which did not, but they judged the GID boys as looking "less all-boy," "less masculine" and "less rugged," but "more handsome" than the other boys. The GID girls were judged as looking "more masculine," "more rugged," "more tomboyish" and "more handsome" than other girls.

All transsexuals have sexual identities at odds with their bodies, but in addition, both the men and the women have a variety of sexual orientations. A transsexual man or woman can be straight, gay, bisexual or asexual (experiencing no sexual attraction), so it's obvious that whatever underlies their sexual identity is not the same as what underlies their sexual orientation. This can get quite confusing: a transsexual woman may feel like a man and also love men; surgery converts her female body to that of a man but her *brain* is that of a gay male, not a straight one. The opposite of that also occurs: a male transsexual feels like a woman but also loves women; surgery converts his body to a female one, but her brain is that of a lesbian, not a heterosexual woman.

In the Netherlands, where more data on transsexuals has been gathered, it's estimated that 60 percent of male-to-females are attracted to men and 10 percent are bisexual. About 95 percent of female-to-males are attracted to women. (They may have been living as lesbians before.) Among the small minority of female-to-males who are attracted to men are people like David Harrison, whose story follows.

HOW CATHERINE BECAME DAVID

David Harrison is a 44-year-old playwright and actor who lives in New York. I interviewed him by telephone. He spoke with a soft English accent, a carry-over from his early life in England, where he lived until he was twelve years old and his concert pianist father moved the family to Canada.

In those days David was known as Catherine, elder sister to two brothers and a younger sister. He describes himself as a shy child with few close relationships. Alone in the attic, Catherine would spend hours reading history books or dressing up as Peter Pan and other male characters from books, plays, television and film. She had fantasies about the Beatles: Paul and George having sex with one another, Catherine taking turns being one or the other.

David recalls that he, as Catherine, always felt like a boy. When she was only five, Catherine asked her mother if she could change into a boy. Her mother, an artistic woman with liberal attitudes, allowed Catherine to have short hair and dress in pants at home. But at school Catherine had no choice. She hated wearing the girls' school uniform and being confined to the girls' playground. Her preferred playmates were boys and, though she disliked rough play, she preferred boyish activities like soccer over the usual girls' games. The arrival of puberty was a nightmare for Catherine. She despised her developing female body, became quite depressed and gained a lot of weight. She felt that "now there is no way out."

The move to Canada felt like a reprieve. David recalls Catherine's excitement about being able to start a new life where nobody knew her. Away from the school uniforms and the enforced "girls only" playground of England, Catherine became more outgoing. A bright student, at age 17 she represented her high school on a Canadian TV quiz show called "Reach for the Top" and came third in Canada. At the same time, she avoided the whole high school dating scene. Her one major "crush" was on a girlfriend who later came out as a lesbian.

When Catherine was 19 she declared herself a lesbian, though "part of me felt I was coming out as a gay man," David says now. He recalls "living vicariously" through the sexual escapades of a gay friend. For awhile Catherine worked as a female dominatrix. "It was wonderful having men worshipping me," David recalls, "but even though I was dressed in female drag, inside I actually felt like a gay man tricking."

Then, in her early 30s, Catherine became involved with Kate Bornstein, a well-known playwright, actor and author of a book — *Gender Outlaw* — that's become the rage in Gender Studies courses. Kate is a male-to-female transsexual who, after three marriages, at age 37 underwent a gender change and became a woman, but a gay woman. She and Catherine were together three years when Catherine, at age 35, decided to go through a gender change herself. "What happened," says David now, "is that Kate made it safe for me to look at my gender. I always knew I'd had gender issues, but I was never able to deal with them until Kate. She's a wonderful, supportive person and we're still very close."

Ironically, Kate's encouragement of Catherine to resolve her gender confusion ended up costing her their relationship. Catherine began treatment with male hormones and after a year completely lost interest in sex with women. She changed her name to David and began dating men. "It felt wonderful, being wanted — as a man, by other men," David recalls. He is one of the female-to-male transsexuals who have declined genital surgery. "Although I'd love to have the 'right' equipment," he says, "the technology isn't here yet and I'm not holding my breath. I really do have most of what I want and (for me) the rest is about acceptance. I'm happy to be exactly who I am — a man with different plumbing from other men."

Looking back on his life, David says, "When I hit puberty, something stopped. I didn't grow up. I couldn't, because I was living in the wrong gender. It wasn't until I'd started receiving male hormones, moved out to live on my own, and began living as a man dating other men, that I finally felt like an adult."

How did other people react to the new David? "Mostly fine," he says, "though two lesbian friends couldn't handle it. They may have felt I was 'selling out.'" As David's mother had died when he was 19, she did not see his transition. His father found David's gender change difficult, but said he wasn't altogether surprised by it, and he sees David as being happier and much more relaxed now. David's two younger brothers seem to have accepted it, but his sister Lucy, a lesbian, initially felt betrayed. "I think of him now as a kind of third sex," she says. "But I have to admit that David and I now get along better than Catherine and I ever did."

At age 45, David appears to be a contented man. "I'm not covering up my essence any more," he told me. He loves New York and he loves his work. He continues to tour his "partly autobiographical" solo play, FTM (female-to-male), which he has performed at theatre festivals and colleges. He lives alone, which he prefers, but has a (non-monogamous) committed relationship with a man he describes as "a real soulmate."

The different gender-change outcomes for David and for his former partner, Kate, exemplify the fact that an individual's gender identity and sexual orientation need not be consistent. In non-transsexuals, both men and women may be either heterosexual or homosexual. Similarly, in transsexuals, both male-to-females and female-to-males may be erotically oriented toward either men or women. Kate Bornstein was originally a man who loved women; after her gender change, she was a woman but still loved women. Her body and social role changed from male to female, but her erotic orientation remained the same. David Harrison was a woman who apparently loved other women; after his gender change, he was a man who loved other men. At first glance, it looks as though David changed his erotic orientation as well as his gender, but I don't believe David ever truly identified inwardly as a female. He himself says that he never really thought of himself as a female and that's why "being a lesbian didn't really fit" for him. I think David's true identity and erotic orientation were always those of a gay male. His life as a lesbian was just one step in his process of getting to where he really belonged.

Despite the terrible stress that transsexuals endure in growing up feeling they're in the wrong body, most of them do not develop symptoms of mental disorder. Many of those who seek treatment at gender-change clinics have been married, had children and tried to comply with societal expectations. Eventually they have given up the fruitless struggle of trying to be straight, and have begun pursuing their own destiny. Male transsexuals often delay their reassignment to the female sex until the children are grown. (Children do not become transsexuals because they were raised by transsexual parents, just as children raised by homosexual parents have no greater chance of becoming gay than do children raised by heterosexual parents.)

Because most transsexuals recall experiencing a high level of personal stress while growing up, and many of them also report a history of family strain and disruption, some sociologists have concluded that family dynamics were the cause of the transsexualism. I believe it's more plausible that these families, rather than *causing* the child's transsexualism, were responding negatively to their child's conviction of being in the wrong sex. It's highly likely that most parents, knowing nothing about gender identity disorder or transsexualism, would be upset if their little son insists he's a girl, adores Barbie dolls, hates cars and trucks, and likes to play dress-up (as a "lady," of course) long after other little boys have abandoned dress-ups for soccer.

There's no good evidence that transsexualism is caused by home environment, just as there's no good evidence that certain home environments produce other sexual types. Almost all transsexuals report feeling they were simply born different. The female-to-male transsexuals studied by sociologist Holly Devor were "nearly unanimous in their assertions that, whatever other influences later came to bear, they were born as women who were destined to become men."

According to historical accounts, transsexuality around the world has always existed, but it's only since the last half of the 20th century that efforts have been made to identify it and offer treatment to those who want it. It used to be believed that male-to-female transsexuals outnumbered female-to-males by about three to one, based on the fact that many more men than women present themselves to gender dysphoria clinics. However, clinicians are now speculating that transsexualism may occur equally in men and women but fewer women seek treatment. Maybe that's because it's easier for women to live as men than it is for men to live as women. Women can disguise their sex in male clothes and male haircuts, but men cannot disguise their deep voices, their facial hair and their muscular builds under female clothing and hairstyles.

How many transsexuals are there? In the Netherlands it is known that there is one male-to-female transsexual per 11,900 men, and one female-to-male transsexual per 30,400 women. Elsewhere it's been estimated that one in 30,000 people is born transsexual, which would mean about 1,000 in Canada and 10,000 in the United States. It's beginning to look as though these numbers are probably too low, though, as the numbers of transsexuals appear to be increasing worldwide. It's anybody's guess whether this means an actual increase in the incidence of transsexuality or merely an increase in the number of transsexuals who are "coming out." Certainly more transsexuals than ever before are going public with their stories.

For many transsexuals, the desire to be physically transformed has little or nothing to do with their desire to have sex. In fact, many transsexuals appear to be undersexed; they are content to take medications that abolish sexual arousal completely.

MAKING A WOMAN OUT OF A MAN, AND VICE VERSA

The first transsexual to receive worldwide publicity was Christine Jorgensen, who became famous when she revealed that she was formerly George, an ex-G.I. from New York. Although Jorgensen was not the first person to have a surgical sex change, she was the first to become famous for doing so. In 1951, shy 26-year-old George had travelled to Copenhagen for surgery to transform his body to female. A year later, instead of George it was Christine Jorgensen who returned to the U.S. I remember when the news of this flashed around the world: the primary reaction was one of amusement and the second reaction was derision. Very few people, including doctors, knew anything about transsexualism in the 1950s. Christine Jorgenson was regarded by most people as a silly, confused man. People wondered why doctors would agree to do such ridiculous surgery.

It was not until two decades later that the first sex-change operation in America took place, at the University of Minnesota. Richard Raskin, a physician and tennis star who had married and had a son, became Renee Richards. (Her past was exposed when she was initially prohibited from competing as a woman in the professional tennis circuit.) Another American celebrity, electronic music pioneer Walter Carlos, also became a pioneer in sex change when he became Wendy Carlos. In Britain, newspaperman James Morris, who had climbed Mount Everest in 1953, became female travel writer Jan Morris.

Such famous cases sparked widespread interest among transsexuals all over the world. Soon dozens of them, in many countries, came to the attention of the medical profession. As the numbers increased, the need for official standards of care became obvious. These were finally created in the late 1970s by the International Dysphoria

Symposium; gender dysphoria clinics around the world are expected to adhere to these standards.

The gender clinic I know best is the one in Vancouver — a publicly funded clinic at Vancouver General Hospital known as the B.C. Centre for Sexual Medicine, where 70 to 90 people a year seek treatment for gender dysphoria. It's one of only two such clinics in Canada (the other is in Montreal). The information that follows concerning the treatment of transsexuals at these clinics is based on information provided by the Vancouver clinic.

A person must be referred to the clinic by a physician or mental health team, but because of the demand, it can take many months to set up the initial assessment. The assessment begins with the applicant being seen by two senior clinicians who have not discussed the case with one another beforehand. The patient also completes a series of questionnaires. On the basis of all this information, the clinic's team develops recommendations for hormone therapy and possibly for personal therapies including counselling, family therapy and speech coaching. (Discussion of surgery will come later if the patient decides to proceed to that.)

The hormonal treatment of transsexual male-to-females has two main objectives: to reduce the amount of testosterone produced by the testicles, and to help the person develop female body characterisics. (Unfortunately, not much can be done about the broader shoulders and slimmer hips typical of men.) Giving the person estrogen and progesterone reduces the production of testosterone and helps to develop female characteristics including softer skin, less beard, less body hair, more breast development and female fat distribution to the thighs, buttocks and abdomen. These changes sometimes take years to come about. Breast development takes at least six years and the process cannot be hurried by taking hormone doses higher than those typically produced by the female body. Hair growth on face and body is difficult to change as, after a person has experienced years of testosterone action, even very small amounts of testosterone can cause continued facial and body hair growth. Patients frequently seek electrolysis for the problem. Unfortunately, the deep male voice remains despite the other feminizing changes that take place. That's because the voice breaking in puberty is due to growth of the larynx and that produces an irreversible change in the voice.

Female-to-male transsexuals are put on an opposite schedule. Testosterone injections produce masculinization, including an enlarged clitoris, the growth of facial hair and a typically male distribution of body hair. Frequently the injections also produce male-pattern baldness, so that a woman with gorgeous tresses can end up as a bald man. The muscle bulk increases and this, plus a suitable exercise regime, enables patients to build their upper body muscle development into a more masculine shape. At high enough doses, testosterone will cause the voice to break and become masculine; once this occurs, the voice change is permanent.

Following hormone therapy, if the person opts to proceed to sex-change surgery, he must first complete a minimum one-year "real-life test," which involves a full year of supervised complete immersion in the role of the chosen sex. (Some clinics in Britain and elsewhere require a two-year test). During this time the person dresses like the desired sex, assumes a new name and tells her family, friends and employer of the new identity and the plans for surgery.

How many people go on to have surgery? That's difficult to say because the time lag between seeking treatment at the clinic and having surgery can be huge. "For example," Blaine Beemer of the Vancouver clinic told me, "a patient who came to us ten years ago has only now decided to have surgery." Beemer also pointed out that many people who present themselves for treatment are not transsexual at all; they have psychological problems and mistakenly believe that changing their sex will alleviate their unhappiness. What these people need, he said, is psychological help, not hormone treatment and surgery.

Among the true transsexuals, those who decide to have their sexual organs altered must travel to the Montreal clinic, where about 200 operations a year are performed, or to clinics in the U.S. and Europe.

The United States has several university-based sexology clinics, the best known of which is the University of Minnesota's Center for Sexual Health, which has offered a comprehensive range of sexual health services for more than three decades and is internationally regarded. Transsexual people there receive a range of services similar to those provided at the Vancouver clinic. Most people, of course, do not have access to such comprehensive clinics as those in Vancouver and Minneapolis. Instead, they must consult various physicians and medical specialists in private practice concerning the different aspects of their therapy and surgery.

Surgery to make a woman's body out of a man's usually includes having breast implants and sometimes building a vagina from the penis or part of the colon. (Many patients decide to forego surgery to construct a vagina; they are content to retain their penis and look like a woman in most other respects.) For those who do have vaginal surgery, a temporary post-surgical stent (a tube-like support) is inserted into the new vagina and then the patient must for several months do twice-daily dilatations at home to prevent the vagina from closing. With no uterus and no ovaries, the person can never become pregnant.

Making a man's body out of a woman's is more difficult. Removing the internal female organs by hysterectomy and removing the breasts by mastectomy are fairly straightforward operations, and many patients don't go beyond that. The small number who wish to go on to phalloplasty (surgically building a penis) soon learn that it is very difficult to create a penis that looks authentic and that also enables the person to urinate in the male standing position so that he can pass as a man in men's washrooms. Some transsexuals also want to be able to have penetrative intercourse. Pioneering work by plastic surgeons in the Netherlands has gone a long way toward meeting these requirements — for example, creating a penis from a flap taken from the arm, and using a variety of stiffening prostheses — but the results are still far from perfect. At the Montreal clinic, it takes two surgeons about seven hours to remove skin from the patient's forearm and use it to construct a penis. Even with a workable penis, however, the person can never father children, as there are no testicles to produce sperm and no ducts to carry the sperm to the urethra.

In Canada most provinces pay for hormonal treatments and some surgeries. For example, transsexuals requesting breast enlargement are treated the same as biological women who require it. About half of the provinces pay for genital sex-change surgeries if they are performed at the Montreal clinic or in a handful of approved clinics in Europe and the U.S.

In places where such surgery is not covered by a public health plan, the costs can be very steep indeed. But despite the huge financial burden, thousands of men and women in North America and Europe, desperate to be changed into their "real" bodies, have now undergone sex-change treatments. Many of them have worked and saved for years; when one surgical procedure is paid for, they begin saving for the next one.

A few years ago the Canadian Department of Defence surprised everyone by paying for a soldier, Sergeant Sylvain Durand, to change his sex. (Newspapers across the country noted how much the Canadian military had changed since the time, not too long ago, when revealing any non-heterosexual identity was enough to bring a dishonourable discharge.) Sergeant Durand's story was chronicled in a Life Network TV documentary, *Yale Island Transsexuals*, about people undergoing sex-change operations at the Montreal clinic.

Born a biological male, Durand had tried hard to fulfill his expected role: he married, fathered two children, even joined the army in a bid to become a "real" man. But nothing he did could cure his unhappiness. Finally, after seeing a psychiatrist, he gained the courage to proceed with a sex change to become "Sylvie."

Female hormones redistributed Sylvie's fat to a female form and softened her skin. Her mammary glands developed — "like a teenager," she recalled. The most difficult hurdle was making her beard disappear, which took a year of painful laser treatments. After the removal of her penis and testicles and the construction of a vagina, she was ecstatic: "It feels like the end of a nightmare," said a tearful and joyous Sylvie. She had by then formed a lesbian relationship with Cynthia, a woman who'd been a Toronto police officer for 28 years before reading about Sylvie's case and gaining the courage to finally admit he was transsexual.

Germaine Greer argues in *The Whole Woman* that, unless you have a womb, you cannot know what it's like to be a woman. But transsexuals like Sylvie clearly illustrate that feeling female doesn't require a female body, let alone a womb. People like Sylvie felt female even when they lived in a male body. After surgery, they still feel female although they have no uterus or ovaries. For these women, what's important is having their appearance match their inner female identity and womanly feelings. What brings them happiness is finally being seen by others as the women they've felt like all along. "It's like taking off a mask," one woman said to me after her transition. "At last I'm allowed to live the way I should have been living all my life." Clearly, for these women having a womb is a low priority.

TREATMENT OUTCOMES

Despite the difficulties in female-to-male surgery, follow-up indicates they are somewhat more satisfied with the outcome than are male-to-female transsexuals, though the latter also report a high degree of satisfaction. Dutch researchers did structured interviews of a large number of post-surgical transsexuals, asking them whether they were employed, had partners, were accepted by families, were satisfied with their sex lives and so on. Ninety-seven percent of female-to-male transsexuals and 86 percent of male-to-female transsexuals were satisfied; none of them regretted the decision to undergo sex reassignment. These figures are impressive, especially considering the fact that, after surgery, these people can never produce biological children.

When German researchers compared post-operative male-to-female transsexuals to straight men and women in terms of their self-esteem and certain personality traits, they found that both the transsexuals and straight men had better self-esteem than the straight women (probably due to the "male privilege" enjoyed by both groups as they grew into adulthood). In terms of personality traits, the transsexuals were more androgynous than both other groups — that is, they were intermediate between straight men and women. They were similar to straight men in self-esteem and dynamic body image, but similar to women in typically feminine traits.

American psychologist Richard Lippa compared transsexuals to straight people in terms of their occupational and hobby preferences, as well as in how masculine or feminine they felt. He found that male-to-female transsexuals were very different from straight men in terms of their work and hobby preferences, and they also felt much more feminine than straight men did. Female-to-male transsexuals were very different from their straight sisters in work and hobby preferences, and they felt more masculine than straight women did. However, they were not different from the straight women in "feminine" characteristics related to being people-oriented and expressive. Interestingly, the traits that distinguished transsexuals from straight people were very similar to the traits that distinguished straight men from straight women.

It may surprise readers to know that most transsexuals have little difficulty forming successful long-term sexual relationships following their reassignment. Two-thirds of the female-to-male transsexuals studied by Professor Holly Devor reported that they were romantically and sexually involved. (Incidentally, Holly Devor, who is now the Dean of Graduate Studies at the University of Victoria, at age 50 became Aaron Devor, abandoning his life as a masculine lesbian and assuming a new identity as a man.)

One female-to-male transsexual who has established a successful long-term relationship, despite his decision not to have phalloplasty, was reported by psychiatrist Lynne Webster in the *British Journal of Sexual Medicine*:

John is a junior partner in a prestigious firm of accountants, with a promising future career. Only the senior partner knows that John was born female, and underwent gender change between university and his clerkship. This was a carefully planned transition after psychological assessment and hormonal masculinization. A hysterectomy and mastectomies were timed not to interfere with his exams. He decided against phalloplasty with the full support of his long-term female partner, a legal secretary. They are now the proud parents of a baby daughter conceived by artificial insemination. It is an abiding regret for John that his parents have not been able to accept the transition, but he has no other regrets about his choice and he hopes that with the arrival of a grandchild, their attitude will soften.

A few years ago Jack Johnston, who'd been teaching Grade 5 at Henderson Elementary School in Vancouver for eight years, took a medical leave and returned to school after the Christmas break with his identity legally and medically changed to that of a woman, Jenna Stuart. Ms. Stuart was greeted with a round of applause from the students, who had been prepared for the change by the school's principal. She reported that the students had been quite accepting of the change, but they'd wanted to know if their teacher would wear a dress now and whether she would still be taking them on the expected field trip to Lynn Valley Canyon. Most of the parents (who were informed of the change and were offered new school placements for their children if desired) were also accepting; only six families had their children moved to new schools.

Sexual transition of the oldest person I know of occurred in Victoria, B.C., in 2003. Arnell Smith, a former corporal in the Royal Air Force, father of two, grandfather of 10, great-grandfather of 11, started living as a woman, Frances Smith, at the age of 81. She'd been married to Grace for 58 years. Speaking to newspaper reporter Gwendolyn Richards, Frances recalled a childhood filled with longing to play with girls, sneaking girl clothes from a sister's closet, later buying herself (then himself) satin and lace underwear. Fifteen years ago she got a computer and discovered on the internet that there were many others like herself. She'd been cross-dressing on weekends for several years, with Grace's okay. Now, with hormone treatments, she grew breasts. When she finally made the decision to "come out" fully as a woman, she delivered notes to her neighbours in the trailer park, informing them that they might notice another woman (her) coming and going from the Smith home. Most of the family have accepted Frances' transition. She attends two support groups for transsexuals in Victoria. She contemplated sex-change surgery but was warned it was medically risky at her age. "I'd like to have the operation," she told reporter Richards, "but I have to think of Grace."

Despite such apparent successes in their new lives, most transsexuals still encounter many difficulties after their transitions, including the problem of which public washroom to use, which is particularly difficult for those who are pre-surgical. Rather than simply enforcing the transsexual employee's right to use the washroom that he/she feels is appropriate, some employers have gone to great lengths to find a separate washroom so that other employees do not have to share their washrooms with a transsexual co-worker. That may not be necessary: Gail Owen, a human rights advocate for her

Public Service Alliance union in British Columbia, finds that, after about a month, co-workers lose interest in which washroom a trans-sexual uses.

The B.C. Human Rights Tribunal ruled in 2001 that transsexuals have the right to use the washroom of their choice, and that for all human rights matters, transsexuals should be considered to be members of their desired sex whether or not they have had surgery to alter their biological sex. The ruling was in response to a complaint by a pre-surgery transsexual, Tawni Sheridan, who was threatened with eviction in a nightclub where she used the women's washroom.

Sadly, there is still a great deal of prejudice against transsexual people, even among people who accept other sexual minorities. I think part of the problem is that transsexuality is uncommon: most people have never known a transsexual and so they tend to think of them in "drag queen" stereotypes. To many people the very idea of changing into another sex seems preposterous; it makes them feel uncomfortable and anxious, or else irritated and angry. It probably doesn't help that transsexuals, especially early in the transition process, tend to exaggerate their feminine or masculine dress and appearance, making themselves look like parodies of women or men instead of the real thing. Even when a male-to-female trans-sexual does not overdress, the broad shoulders, slim hips and deep male voice coming from an apparent female can be surprising, if not unnerving, for people who know little or nothing about transsexualism.

Many transsexuals lose their jobs, their partners, their children, their families and friends. This is especially true of the male-to-females, who tend to be older than the female-to-males and more likely to have been married with children and therefore have more to lose in terms of family relationship. Often they are forced to move away and become socially isolated. In addition, they begin to experience the same discrimination that other women complain of. They report that, after they become women, the plumbers, repairmen and auto mechanics they deal with regard them as less competent; consequently, they begin to *feel* less competent than they did as men. They also become more self-conscious about their appearance and their weight. Though they want to find partners, they tend to be looking more for friendship and love than for sex, which is a problem for most of the men they meet. They have difficulty finding and keeping employment too, despite the fact that, on average, they have more education than others. Job dissatisfaction is high among them, as the "female" jobs they find pay much less than the "male" jobs they held formerly.

With female-to-male transsexuals the situation is quite different. Their gender transition is easier because women who dress as men are simply more acceptable in society than men who dress as women. Also, they can "pass" more easily in their new gender because their voices and body forms are less incongruous. They begin, for the first time in their lives, to enjoy the privileges that still accrue to men in our society. They are often able to obtain better-paid employment than they were as women and to experience more personal power. On the other hand, as Holly Devor reported, many of them came "to understand that in forfeiting their womanhood they had also cut themselves off from the warmth and emotional vitality of women's companionship ... they had to satisfy themselves with men's rough and competitive camaraderie, which, more often than not, left them painfully cold."

Intersexuals

Is it a boy or a girl? That's the first thing people ask when a baby's born. But occasionally neither the doctor nor the parents can answer the question. That's because the baby's been born with ambiguous genitals and internal organs that make it difficult to say whether the child is male or female. Sometimes the erectile tissue has an unusual shape or size, so that the doctor or midwife cannot say whether it is a penis or a clitoris. Sometimes the tissue forming the penis hasn't fused properly, and the urethra may not open at the end of the penis, as expected, but at some other place. The baby's labia may be partially fused, making it difficult to distinguish it from a scrotum that's empty and split instead of fused. The infant's testicles may be undescended or completely absent. Or the child may be born with a uterus and a penis. Once in a while the child's gonads may each be a combination of ovary and testicle, or else the child may have one ovary and one testicle. Sometimes the shape of the genitals may not correspond to the child's chromosomal sex. The cause of all these anomalies can be hormonal or chromosomal.

These babies were previously known as "hermaphrodites," from the names of the Greek gods Hermes and Aphrodite. According to Greek mythology, their child, Hermaphroditus, fell in love and was fused with a male nymph, becoming half male and half female. Today babies with both male and female sexual features are called "intersexuals," meaning "between sexes."

Estimates of how many people are born intersexual vary in different countries because the frequency of the relevant genes varies around the world. When researchers from Brown University surveyed the medical literature from 1955 to 2000 they concluded that as many as two percent of live births may be intersexual in some way — that is, in their chromosomes, gonads, genitals or hormones. They also concluded that "corrective" genital surgery on these infants probably runs between one or two per thousand live births.

The arrival of an intersex child typically throws the parents into a panic. If the doctor can't say whether the child is a boy or a girl, the parents will probably see their baby's ambiguous genitalia as evidence that the child is "abnormal," "a freak." And in fact, the condition used to be regarded as so shameful that parents were advised never to tell their children about their condition. Thankfully, those days are gone, but it's only very recently that doctors have begun resisting the temptation to surgically "correct" these infants.

Sometimes an intersex infant has a condition that threatens its life or its bodily functioning. For example, if the child lacks a urethra, a doctor must operate at once to save its life. Most of the time, however, the physician knows that the intersex condition is not a threat to the infant's life or health; the baby may have a perfectly healthy body but with genitals that look different from other people's.

Nevertheless, modern medicine has not regarded these infants as just another normal sexual variant, but as a social and psychological emergency, based on the belief that only rapid intervention would avoid psychological and social problems later on.

Therefore, the standard medical response has been (and still is, in many places) to inform the parents that there is a problem and that it requires immediate action to "fix" it. The frightened parents typically accede, and the doctors proceed with plans to "correct" the infant's appearance so that it will look more "normal."

About 90 percent of intersexed babies who are surgically "corrected" are altered to be females, regardless of their genetic sex. That's because it's easier to construct a vagina than a satisfactory penis. Typically, the baby's phallus was measured. If it was longer than 2.5 cm, the child was usually treated as a boy, even when it was genetically female; if the phallus was shorter than 2.5 cm, usually the mini-penis was cut off, the child was castrated and treated as a female. Any clitoris 1 cm or longer was usually reduced in size, even though this could impair the individual's sexual pleasure.

What is the medical rationale for these surgeries? Doctors have claimed that, if left unaltered, these babies would suffer irreparable psychological and social trauma. But in fact, there is no compelling evidence to support this contention. There is no evidence that intersexual babies in the past who were *not* surgically altered turned out to have more psychological or social problems than those born more recently who underwent surgery and hormonal treatments. Anne Fausto-Sterling, Professor of Biology and Women's Studies at Brown

University, reviewed 70 case studies of adolescents and adults who grew up with obviously anomalous genitalia. Quoted in Phyllis Burke's 1996 book, *Gender Shock*, Fausto-Sterling commented, "Almost without exception, these ... children ... grew up knowing they were intersexual (though they did not advertise it) and adjusted to their unusual status ... there is not a psychotic or a suicide in the lot."

How about the psychological effects of surgery on intersexual infants? There is very little scientific information about that, and what little there is, is not reassuring. A 1998 study by a Dutch team reported a high incidence of psychological problems in the surgically altered intersexed children they studied. These were 59 children referred to the Sophia Children's Hospital between 1984 and 1994. Female sex was assigned in infancy to 54 of them, and male sex to five. The children received correction of their genitalia, and (later) counselling. The parents received intensive and long-term counselling. Despite these measures, 39 percent of the children developed severe psychopathology and another 19 percent "mild" psychological problems.

HOW DANNY BECAME DANIELLE

One intersexual baby who was not surgically altered was Danielle Anderson, now a 42-year-old Vancouver woman who calls herself transsexual but was actually born intersexual, with a micropenis, no scrotum and no internal sex organs. Though the hospital recorded her as "Female?" she was raised as a boy. Now a petite, soft-spoken woman with a cloud of shoulder-length curls, she came to our interview dressed in casually fashionable feminine clothing — a cropped top, soft jacket and long jean skirt open at the lower front to reveal shapely legs clad in pantyhose. Her voice is huskier than most women's but not as deep as most men's. She moves, sits and converses like any ordinary woman, but her presentation is somehow more careful, more deliberately feminine.

Though Danielle looks womanly, her history is very different from that of most other women. Her three sisters grew up knowing her as their older brother, "Danny," who often looked after them when they were young, after the parents separated and the mother was out working. From an early age, however, Danny knew she was no ordinary boy. She was expected to play boy games that didn't interest her, but she was not accepted into girls' games that did interest her. Kids at school called her "sexless" and bullied her in gym class. "I was the school punching bag," she recalls. "Nobody liked the kind of boy I was." When she was 12 or 13, boys the same age were becoming interested in girls, but Danny realized she didn't think and relate the way they did; she was sexually attracted to boys.

Not only did she think differently from other boys, as an adolescent she failed to develop a male appearance. Without testes, her own body could not produce the testosterone needed to masculinize her voice and body, so Danny was given injections to help her "become a man." The hormone injections made her voice deepen and eventually she grew a little facial hair, but they did little to change her bodily shape. Their main effect was to make her feel "mean and angry" while having no effect on her inward identity. "I knew the testosterone was all wrong for me," she says now. "Inside I felt female. In movies I related to the female characters, not the male ones. I could understand what the female stars were experiencing because inside I was one of them."

Why didn't she speak out then? Why didn't she protest the attempts to make her more manly? "Because I wasn't raised in an environment where I could talk about my feelings and people would listen," she says now. "I didn't have enough faith in my own thoughts and feelings. Other people seemed confident about what they were doing, so I just went along with what they decided for me." (She deeply regrets that passivity now, knowing that if she had been able to refuse the hormone treatments, she would never have acquired the low voice that is now permanently hers.)

At age 19, Danny had her first sexual experience with a woman who pursued her at work. "I didn't have any feelings for her, but I knew that dating women was what I was supposed to do." Not surprisingly, the experience was unsatisfactory for both of them. Finally, at age 21, Danny quit trying to be a typical man. She decided she must be gay, and for the next 14 years she adopted the role of a gay man. She went to work as a home care worker and loved it. She became involved in the drag queen community. "I never dressed as a woman at home," she says, "but the drag community gave me an acceptable venue to let myself out, which was wonderful. I didn't like being on stage as a drag queen, though. That wasn't what I wanted." But living the rest of her life as a gay man wasn't what she wanted either. "Inside, I knew I felt like a woman, not like a gay man, but I didn't know what to do about it. I didn't even have the language for it; I only knew that I felt constant frustration because the inside me didn't match the outside one."

Then, at the age of 35, Danny heard about the Gender Dysphoria Clinic (now the Centre for Sexual Medicine) in her city. "I had no idea there was such a thing as 'gender dysphoria,'" she says now. A light went on in her brain; at long last, she screwed up her courage to seek counselling at the clinic. By that time she had been in an eight-year live-in relationship with Jim, whom she describes as being "a wonderful man who's 100 percent gay." Danny was terrified of losing Jim if she became Danielle, but she was determined to take that chance.

Eventually Jim was able to accept the transition. Their relationship had always been non-monogamous, now it became non-sexual, too. Danielle says they remain "best friends and loving companions in a committed relationship" who accept the fact that Jim dates gay men while Danielle now dates straight men. "He loves me for *who* I am, not *what* I am," says Danielle.

At the time of our interviews, Danielle had undergone feminizing hormone treatments at the gender dysphoria clinic and had been dressing as a woman for about five years. Unlike many others who change gender, she was fortunate to have family and friends who were able to accept her new persona with little or no fuss. She was pleased to discover that she and her mother had more in common now that they have a "mother/daughter" relationship that includes talking about recipes and shopping for clothes together.

Danielle recalls that the hardest challenge of all for her was "coming out" in female garb at her church. "It's one thing to tell your family and close friends," she says, "but how do you announce to 400 people in your church congregation that you're actually not the person they thought you were?" Eventually she discussed the problem with her pastor, who promised to support her. She's not sure what went on behind the scenes, but when she finally did appear in church dressed as a woman, "nobody batted an eyelash."

Being "out" as a woman hasn't all been smooth sailing, though. Danielle began to receive unwanted attention from men, some of it intended to be positive and some negative. Once her purse was snatched; another time she became the object of a relentless stalker. She learned that she could no longer walk alone at night. Always a poor sleeper, Danny had been in the habit of taking long walks when she couldn't sleep, but when Danny became Danielle, out at night in female garb, a man attacked her and knocked her down. Though she managed to escape, it was a shock realizing that she was now a target.

Despite such difficulties, Danielle reports being much happier "now that I can be who I really was all along. For the first time in my life, that core of melancholy is gone." Her experience as a woman continues to broaden. When I interviewed her, she was thrilled to have been invited recently to her first all-female baby shower. Most importantly, following our interview she completed surgery to construct a vagina. "Finally my outside and inside match," says Danielle.

The practice of surgically altering intersexual newborns is a fairly recent one. In earlier times, infants with ambiguous genitalia were simply accepted. In some cultures — the Chinese, for example — they were regarded as good luck omens. The Jewish Talmud a thousand years ago laid down rules guiding the respect and treatment of intersex persons. In western countries in earlier times intersexuals had to choose whether to live as men or women, but there was no attempt to physically alter them. Until the 1950s, that is, when psychologist John Money, along with psychiatrists Joan and John Hampson (all of them at Johns Hopkins University), developed case-management principles for treating intersex infants. These principles were to assign a sex to the child, do the surgery and shield the parents from the terrible knowledge that their child had ambiguous genitalia. The principles were based on Money's (mistaken) belief that sexual identity is completely malleable for the first 18 months of life.

THE "JOHN/JOAN" CASE

The doctors' belief that they were doing the right thing was strengthened by the favourable publicity about such cases reported by Money and the Hampsons. In Money's 1972 book *Man & Woman, Boy & Girl*, he described the now-famous "John/Joan" case — the case of a genetically identical male twin, Bruce Reimer of Winnipeg, whose penis was ablated when he was eight months old, in a botched cautery operation for a tight foreskin. Money advised the parents to raise the child as a girl and arranged to see them and the child for yearly visits to Johns Hopkins Hospital. Bruce was renamed Brenda. Within a year the child had his testicles removed to facilitate his feminization.

Subsequent reports conveyed the strong impression that the child was adjusting well to life as a girl, and that the parents also were doing fine with their "daughter." Money claimed that Brenda grew up to be happily feminine. The case was widely publicized as giving strong support to the view that babies' sexual identity is neutral at birth, and that children develop male or female identities as a result of their socialization. This, of course, strengthened the practice of surgical intervention with intersexed infants. Ignoring the child's innate sexual identity, doctors purported to surgically create another one, believing that raising the child as a boy or a girl would ensure that the child felt like an ordinary male or female.

But there were cases, even prior to Money, that challenged this assumption. One of the earliest was reported in a 1934 article published in the *Journal of Orthopsychiatry*. The case involved a boy who had been born with an atypical configuration of his penis and urethra, so he was pronounced to be a girl and was christened Margaret. For 14 years he was dressed and treated in every way as a girl. At age 13, the school doctor discovered that Margaret was not a girl; he was referred to a child guidance clinic when he was just under 14. By then he had a deep, masculine voice, and was urgently demanding that he be allowed to live according to his true sexual identity. Clinic staff who examined him reported that he looked obviously like a boy wearing girls' clothing. He was "masculine in every respect ... there was nothing in his manner, features or appearance that would suggest femininity ... his interests were as nearly those of a healthy adolescent boy as would be possible under the circumstances."

The boy's story was that he had always associated with girls but he had always been regarded as a tomboy. When his voice began to change he began to have sexual feelings for girls. He began having dreams in which he was a boy or a man, never a girl.

He became more and more proficient in typically boy activities. His parents, initially opposed to having him change sex because of the embarrassment it would bring upon them, finally agreed. On his 14th birthday he was "transformed" from Margaret to James at the Child Guidance Clinic. Sporting a short haircut and male clothing, he went directly to a small institution caring for boys and girls, where he could associate with boys as a boy. He was dubbed a sissy at first, but in time his ability in baseball made him into a hero for the younger boys.

James remained in the institution for 20 months. Staff there reported that his social adjustment was so phenomenal, there was never a need for him to receive psychotherapy. Toward the end of his stay, James chose a girlfriend and appeared not to be conflicted about sexual matters. He left the institution and entered a new junior high school, where he was accepted as a boy. James' parents had great difficulty in accepting his transition, and while he was in the institution they completely rejected him as a son. Fortunately, a sympathetic older half-sister and her husband took James under their wing, and when they moved to another city when James was 16, he moved with them. He continued to write to the child guidance clinic staff in his former city, informing them that he was doing fine at school, had made friends with both boys and girls and had been pursuing his athletic interests. In his last year of high school he was quarterback of the high school football team. There is no information about James' life as an adult.

SEXUAL IDENTITY IS INBORN

The "John/Joan" case also challenged the notion that sexual identity is completely malleable at birth. Although touted as a complete success at the time and for two decades afterward, later information revealed a quite different outcome. In 1994, biologist Milton Diamond of Hawaii/Manoa University tracked Brenda down and discovered that in her early 20s she had chosen a sex-change operation back to male. A few years later, Dr. Diamond and Dr. Keith Sigmundson, a Canadian psychiatrist, published an article about the results of their investigation. They had reviewed the medical and clinical notes on the case and noted the impressions of therapists who were originally involved. They had also conducted current interviews with the adult Bruce (renamed David), his mother and others.

The results of their investigation strongly challenged the notion that individuals are psychosexually neutral at birth. The mother reported that treating the child as a girl was a disaster. Brenda had disliked girls' toys and clothes, preferring her brother's toys and boys' activities. By the time she was between nine and 11, it was clear to Brenda herself that she was different. At school she was teased for looking like a boy wearing girls' clothes and for trying to urinate standing up; other children called her "cave girl" and "gorilla." She complained to doctors at Johns Hopkins and also to her local therapists, but apparently her complaints fell on deaf ears. At age 12 Brenda was put on an estrogen regime. She did not want to be more feminine and often threw the hormone away. She was unhappy about getting breasts and refused to wear a bra. She had thoughts of suicide.

Finally, when she was 14, Brenda decided to switch to living as a male named Bruce and refused to return to Johns Hopkins Hospital. The father then told him about the sex reassignment surgery in infancy. Bruce as an adult (renamed David) recalled that moment. "All of a sudden everything clicked. For the first time things made sense and I understood who and what I was." He received male hormone injections and a mastectomy, followed by surgery to construct a penis. When he was 25, he married a women considerably older than himself and adopted her children. (His story, as the adult David Reimer, was chronicled in John Calapinto's book *As Nature Made Him*.)

In the past 15 years, a tidal wave of public protest against hormonal and surgical alteration of intersexuals has arisen. The Intersex Society of North America (ISNA) was founded in 1993 by Cheryl Chase, an intersexual woman in San Francisco who has said she feels betrayed and mutilated and also very angry at doctors who are responsible for such "mutilations." ISNA takes the position that intersexed infants should be left alone to make their own decisions when they are older. The infant's parents should be given information and counselling, and reassured that there is no medical emergency needing immediate action; it is safe to allow the child to grow up and decide for itself what its sexual identity is.

ISNA puts out a newsletter entitled *Hermaphrodites With Attitude*. Supporters have been known to show up at hospitals and try to dissuade doctors from performing surgery on intersexual infants. They tell doctors and others that their own physical and mental health was impaired, rather than being improved, by the surgery they endured during infancy and childhood. A *Vancouver Sun* article by reporter Ian Mulgrew a few years ago included some comments from intersexuals:

> *From David:* "… We are who we are and no amount of surgery and hormones and even conditioning … can change that … What was done to me is legally and scientifically sanctioned traumatic sexual abuse."

> *From Randy:* "… It's okay to be different. The parents should wait until the child, health permitting, reaches a level of maturity so he can decide for himself whether or not to opt for surgery."

> *From Lynn:* "Intersex children should be protected and loved and allowed to assume whichever gender they like … I've met several other hermaphrodites who had surgeries during infancy, and I can tell you that they are miserable …"

Many other intersexuals have reported feeling angry and betrayed, and convinced they have been robbed of their true identity.

CHANGING DOCTORS' ATTITUDES

The American Academy of Pediatrics initially referred to Cheryl Chase and her supporters as "zealots" and refused to let Ms. Chase present the patient's point of view to the Academy members. But in

May 2000, Chase was invited to address the Lawson Wilkins Pediatric Endocrine Society at the close of its Boston symposium on the treatment of genital ambiguity in newborns. Her reception was a strong signal that the medical profession is changing its attitudes about the treatment of intersexuality; in fact, several of those who spoke before Ms. Chase had already urged doctors to abandon the current treatment of intersexed babies and instead give parents and their affected offspring the psychological counselling and other supports they may need to cope with their experience.

Two months after Cheryl Chase's address to the Lawson Wilkins Pediatric Endocrine Society, an article in *Pediatrics*, the official magazine of the American Academy of Pediatrics, cited the famous "Joan/John" case and described an additional case in which a child born XY (male) was raised as a female. In adolescence, the "girl" declared herself a boy, discontinued estrogen therapy, had her breasts (which had developed in response to the estrogen) removed and started testosterone replacement. He stated that, since early childhood, he had felt like "a boy trapped in a girl's body." The mother, who did not recall ever being told her infant was genetically male, reported that she always raised her child as a girl but recalled that he had always "acted like a boy." "In light of the accumulating long-term follow-up data," stated the authors of the article, "whenever possible, reconstructive genital surgery should be delayed until the patient's gender identity can be incorporated into the decision-making process."

The doctors' shift in attitude is just one more sign of the interesting cultural change that's blowing across our sexual landscape, signalling a greater acceptance of the large sexual variety that exists among human beings.

5

Different Brains
for Different Sexualities

Some people may be Rooshans, and others may be
Prooshans; they are born so, and will please
themselves. Them which is of other naturs think
different.

Mrs. Gamp in *Martin Chuzzlewit*, by CHARLES DICKENS

A FTER MY ELDEST SON came out as a gay man,
for the first time in my life I got to know a lot
of gay people. And I made a very interesting
discovery: gay men were not just sexually different from other men;
they were often different in other ways. In certain aspects they
seemed to be more like my women friends than like other men I
knew — sensitive, emotionally expressive, willing to talk about personal things and feelings. But often they had other distinguishing
features, too. They were wittier, more acerbic, more creative, more
interested in the arts, more unconventional in their ideas, than
most of the other men I'd known. They actually seemed to *think*
differently.

How different *are* gay and straight people, apart from their obvious sexual difference? *Do* they think differently? Are their brains

different from one another, as we saw in Chapter 2 that the brains of straight men and women are different?

A number of studies reported in this chapter do report differences between gay and straight brains and thinking patterns, but consistent differences are much more often found in gay men than in lesbian women. As noted earlier, there's been far less research on lesbians than on gay men. And when lesbians have been studied, the differences found between them and straight women are often much smaller (or non-existent) than the differences between gay and straight men. It looks as though the development of homosexuality in females and males may differ in important ways, but we don't yet know enough about that. I think it's likely that the *averages* reported for lesbians are misleading because they're derived from the scores of straight women who call themselves lesbian for political or social reasons, combined with the scores of women whose lesbianism may be biologically determined. This could hide real differences that may actually exist between "biological" lesbians (but not "political" lesbians) and straight women.

In this chapter lesbians are mentioned wherever there is relevant information, but most of the information available, and reported here, concerns gay men.

When reading about differences between gay and straight brains, please remember these are average differences. There's a lot of overlap between gays and straights, just as there is between straight men and women. Many gay people are more like straights in some respects than they are like other gays, and vice versa.

Some people have told me they feel it's risky to point out brain differences between gay and straight people. They're worried that others will interpret the differences as meaning "odd" or "inferior." It's the same argument that's used against talking about differences between men and women. My own belief, as noted in Chapter 2, is that we should be encouraging people to accept differences, rather than pretending they don't exist. Differences are interesting; they give life spice and variety. Surely there can be no single "correct" way to be, whether you're male or female, gay or straight. It would be a pretty dull world if we were all clones. Not only that, but our chances of survival would be diminished. Mother Nature knows that; that's why she thrives on diversity.

GAY BRAINS AND STRAIGHT BRAINS

Two Dutch researchers first reported finding a difference between gay and straight brains. The year was 1990. Working in their lab at the Netherlands Institute for Brain Research, they'd found a tiny cluster of brain cells, the *suprachiasmatic nucleus* (SCN), that was nearly twice as large in the brains of homosexual men (who had died of AIDS) as it was in the brains of the dead heterosexual men they examined. The report made headlines, of course, and it also stimulated a lot of discussion in the scientific community. It was a curious finding, because there don't appear to be any male/female differences in the SCN. The SCN doesn't even seem to be involved with sex; instead, it's the mainspring of the biological clock that generates the body's daily rhythms, including the sleep/wake rhythms. (It's been suggested that the enlarged SCN in homosexuals may relate to the fact that, on average, they naturally sleep less. They awaken earlier and go to sleep later than heterosexuals, and so far nobody knows why. One observer suggested it's because most of them don't have children to tire them out!)

Though the Dutch researchers couldn't say what the SCN difference meant, in a later paper one of them (Dick Swaab) was able to describe how the difference comes about. At birth, he explained, the SCN contains less than 20 percent of its adult cell count. Then it begins to develop rapidly and reaches its full size at 13 to 16 months. In heterosexuals, the cells gradually die off so that in adulthood only about 35 percent of them remain. In homosexuals, however, for some reason the cells do not die off, so the SCN of adult homosexuals has the same peak number of cells found in 13- to 16-month-old infants.

Some people argued that the larger SCN in these gay men's brains might have somehow been related to their having had AIDS. However, when Swaab examined the dead brains of two male-to-female transsexuals who did not suffer from AIDS, he found that they, too, had an enlarged SCN, which persuaded him that it wasn't AIDS that caused the gay men's enlarged SCN.

The year after Swaab published his SCN findings, another bombshell was dropped on the scientific community. Simon LeVay, a young neuroanatomist working at the Salk Institute in California, announced in 1991 that he'd examined a tiny cell cluster, the *third interstitial nucleus of the anterior hypothalamus*, or INAH$_3$, in the hypothalamus. The cluster was in an area (the SDN-POA described in Chapter 2) which had earlier been shown to be smaller in women than in men. Now LeVay found that the INAH$_3$ was more than two times larger in straight men than in gay men (in whom it's about the same size as in women).

LeVay's discovery received an enormous amount of publicity. He also received a lot of criticism, both from those who refused to believe that sexual orientation might be biological, and from those who feared that such information might be used against gays. Some critics argued that the smaller SDN in gay brains may have been caused by the gay men's sexual behaviour rather than being inborn. Others argued that the SDN was smaller in the brains of LeVay's cadavers not because they were gay, but because they'd died of AIDS and the size of the SDN is related to testosterone level, which is known to drop in men with AIDS. However, later research by American research psychiatrist William Byne and others showed that HIV status did not influence the size of the INAH$_3$. Byne's group also confirmed that the volume of INAH$_3$ was smaller in gays not because they had fewer neurons there but because the neurons were more densely packed than they were in straight men. No explanation for this was proposed.

Despite the controversy surrounding LeVay's discovery, similar kinds of findings kept rolling in. In 1992 two neuroscientists at the University of California reported they had found gay/straight differences in the *anterior commissure*, the tract of nerve fibres connecting the two hemispheres at the front of the brain. As noted in Chapter 2, the anterior commissure had been shown to be larger in women than in men. Now the researchers discovered that, in gay men, one part of this area appeared to be "hyperfemale" — that is, it was not only 34 percent larger than in straight men, it was even larger (by 18 percent) than in women. LeVay pointed out that, unlike the SDN, the anterior commissure is not involved in regulating sexual behaviour; therefore its size difference between gays and straights could hardly be attributed to differences in their sexual behaviour as had been claimed regarding the SDN difference. This was simply another difference in brain anatomy related to sexual orientation.

There were more questions than answers, and the following year Melissa Hines of the University of California School of Medicine reported yet another difference, this time in women's brains. Hines had found that one region of the *corpus callosum*, that 10-cm bundle of tightly packed fibres that connects the two cerebral hemispheres, was larger in straight women than in lesbians. (The region was already known to be larger in women than in men.)

What on earth could these findings mean? There was a lot of criticism and speculation, but no firm conclusions. No one could say for sure whether the structural differences in gay brains *caused* sexual orientation or were created in early life along with sexual orientation. While the debate rolled on, discoveries continued to be announced, and they didn't stop with brain anatomy; they went on to include genes. In 1993, medical geneticist Dean Hamer at the U.S. National Cancer Institute announced that his lab had found a gene pattern that was linked to male homosexuality. Media reaction to news of a "gay gene" was explosive, but in fact Hamer never claimed he'd found a gay gene. What he did find was a pattern of five DNA segments (called "markers") in the tip of one arm of the x chromosome (from the mother) that occurred significantly more often in gay men than in others. Of the 40 pairs of gay brothers Hamer studied, 33 shared the same pattern, strongly suggesting that homosexuality could be genetic.

If a trait such as homosexuality is inherited, then two close relatives (such as brothers) should both have the same pattern of markers lying near the gene that underlies that trait. Most of the gay brothers in Hamer's study did share the same pattern of markers, which suggested that their homosexuality might be inherited. If so, what about their other close relatives? Since the gay brothers' pattern of markers was on the x chromosome from the mother, it was more likely that, if any of their male relatives were gay, those relatives would be on the mother's side of the family rather than on the father's. That's exactly what Hamer found: the gay brothers had far more gay uncles and cousins on the mother's side of the family than on the father's side. That finding increased the likelihood that genes were involved in male homosexuality, but whether such genes coded for homosexuality itself, or for some other attribute related to homosexuality, was a mystery. And what about female homosexuality? Hamer's finding occurred only in men and not in the lesbians he studied, so whatever his finding meant was specific to *male* homosexuality.

In 1994, Sandra Witelson of McMaster University announced another difference between gay and straight brains, again in an area of the corpus callosum. The area Witelson studied, known as the *isthmus*, had already been shown to differ in men and women. It had also been shown to be larger in left-handed men (among whom homosexuals are overrepresented.) Now MRI recordings had shown that it was 13 percent larger in gay men than in straight men, a statistically significant difference. Witelson was quoted by medical reporter Paul Taylor in the *Globe and Mail* on November 17, 1994:

"This study has taken the anatomical differences from the middle of the brain [the hypothalamus] up to the cortex, the thinking part of the brain. That's a very big leap ... This is showing that sexual orientation is part of something that is much bigger than just sexual behaviour ... What we are suggesting is that sexual orientation is just one feature in the constellation of characteristics which includes perception and cognitive patterns." In other words, homosexual men appear to have their own unique patterns of thinking, of reasoning, and of mentally apprehending what they observe. In answer to a question about the *meaning* of the size difference in the isthmus, Dr.Witelson said it could produce a different "profile of skills," which might explain why some homosexuals are drawn to certain occupations. It was beginning to look as though there's a lot more to being gay than simply being attracted to the same sex.

BEHAVIOURAL DIFFERENCES BETWEEN GAYS AND STRAIGHTS

All over the world, homosexual men exhibit particular kinds of interests and special skills in certain kinds of occupations. Though gay men are only a small percentage of the population, they are prominent far beyond what their numbers would warrant in all areas requiring creativity and artistic sensitivity, including music, literature, art, architecture and design. It now appears that these talents may be due to differences in how the homosexual brain is structured and functionally organized. For example, homosexuals are more likely than heterosexuals to be left-handed, and left-handedness indicates that the brain's cerebral hemispheres are organized differently from most others. It's long been noted that left-handed people are over-represented in artistic occupations; now it appears that may be because the pool of artistic people contains a large number of homosexuals.

But what has hand preference got to do with anything? Simply this: hand preference — called "handedness" — is one of the best clues as to which hemisphere of the brain handles what kind of information. As noted in Chapter 2, right-handed people almost always process language and other sequential information in the left hemisphere, whereas they use the right hemisphere to process "gestalt" or holistic information such as musical melodies or spatial information. In non-right-handed people, however, the division of labour between the two hemispheres is sometimes arranged differently. This can have an effect on how the person thinks and solves problems.

You may be wondering about the term "non-right-handed." What's wrong with the good old-fashioned "left-handed"? What's wrong is that it doesn't allow for the fact that a large number of people are "mixed-handed." They may write with the left hand but use the right hand for other things such a throwing a ball, brushing teeth, dealing cards or removing the lid from a jar. Similarly, some people may write with their right hand but use their left for other tasks. Both kinds of people are actually mixed in their handedness, regardless of which hand they write with, and this has implications for how their brain is wired. That's why handedness is now measured differently: a "right-handed" person now is a person who consistently prefers to use that hand, including for writing. A "non-right-handed" person prefers the left hand for some things, sometimes (but not always) including writing.

Several studies, from various countries, have reported an increased incidence of non-right-handedness in homosexuals. A review article in 2000 by Kenneth Zucker and associates at the University of Toronto reported that gay men and lesbians were much more likely than straight men and women to be non-right-handed. Gay men had a 34 percent greater chance of being non-right-handed, and lesbians a whopping 91 percent greater chance. These are highly significant differences. The authors arrived at these conclusions after analyzing all the data from 20 studies over the past 50 years that, together, compared handedness in almost 7,000 homosexual men and women and more than 16,000 heterosexual men and women. The results strongly suggest two things: that gay brains are "wired" somewhat differently, and that sexual orientation is laid down in the womb, as hand preference is known to be.

Using the left hand for writing is believed to have one of two causes. It can be genetic — the consequence of having left-handed relatives — or it can result from some developmental deviation from the norm in the womb. Such deviation can cause a variety of other conditions along with the left-handedness. Psychiatrist James Lindesay of Guy's Hospital in London has observed that non-right-handed people are more likely than others to suffer from immune disorders, dyslexia, stuttering, epilepsy, alcoholism, migraine and learning disability. However, they are also more likely than others to be successful in a number of occupations and sports where good visuospatial skills are required, including art, architecture, mathematics, music, tennis and baseball.

To illustrate this point, Dr. Lindesay quotes the biblical Book of Judges, Chapter 20, Verse 16, which reports that the Benjamite army at Gibeah contained "seven hundred chosen men left-handed; every one could sling stones at an hair-breadth, and not miss." Interestingly, says Dr. Lindesay, the men of Gibeah were punished for the same "transgressions" as the Sodomites, suggesting, he says, that even in biblical times left-handedness was associated with homosexuality.

What is the significance of homosexuals being less right-handed than others? Just this: it implies that their brains are organized to process information somewhat differently from others. Dr. Martin Reite at the University of Colorado provided a good example of that when he compared the responses of gay and straight men's brains while they listened to tones played through earphones. He found that straight men showed the typical right hemisphere advantage for processing tones, but in gay men there was no difference in the response of their two hemispheres. Both hemispheres were involved in processing the tones they heard, and that's a pattern more typical of women than of men.

·A similar finding was reported by researchers at McMaster University. They asked gay and straight men wearing earphones to listen to spoken language broadcast to both ears at the same time. Straight men showed the usual left hemisphere advantage for decoding the speech they heard, but gay men showed little or no difference between the two hemispheres, which is the typical case for women. Again, the gay men's brains appeared to be functionally different from those of straight men. It's interesting that both groups were able to do the task accurately, even though they used different brain areas (and perhaps different mental strategies) to do it.

DIFFERENCES IN COGNITIVE ABILITIES

Gay men also have differences in their cognitive abilities — their skills in language, mathematics, music, spatial reasoning and so on. This has nothing to do with intelligence. Three studies of intelligence — one in the 1980s and two in the 1990s — found no overall difference between the IQs of gay and straight men. However, their *pattern* of intellectual abilities was different. One of the studies showed that gay men had higher verbal IQs than straight men and women, and poorer non-verbal IQs, including poorer spatial ability. The second study showed that gay men had higher vocabulary scores than straight men. In the third study, gay men showed greater verbal fluency than that of straight men (both men's groups were still less fluent than the women.)

Researchers in the 1990s, having found that straight men and women differed in verbal and spatial abilities, went on to compare straights and gays in these two areas. It turned out that, in most spatial tests, straight men did better than gay men, who in turn were better than women. When a more difficult kind of spatial test was used (mentally rotating an object in space), gay men did even worse, scoring lower than both gay and straight women.

We can't conclude, however, that gay men's cognitive abilities are simply more "female" than straight men's. In fact, it's now known that homosexual men score in a female direction on tests of only *some* cognitive abilities. In tests of other cognitive abilities they score in a male direction. Sometimes, in fact, they score in an *extremely* male direction. Psychologists Diane Halpern and Marciana Crothers reported that, when tested on cognitive skills other than verbal and spatial skills, or when tested on speed instead of accuracy, gay men are sometimes more different from women than straight men are. For example, on tests of mental rotation *where reaction time is scored*, gay men no longer scored lowest, as they had when only mental rotation was tested. Instead, they now scored in a "super-masculine" direction — that is, they did even better than the straight men, who did better than straight women. The same was true in a test of verbal analogies. But in a test requiring people to generate synonyms for common words, gay men scored lower than both of the straight groups. The researchers concluded from this that homosexuality is associated with its own distinct pattern of cognitive abilities, neither uniformly "male" nor "female." Depending on which particular ability is being measured, homosexuals may score in either direction.

Researchers have also found differences in how gay and straight men think and solve mental problems, just as such differences were found between straight women and men. Psychologists at the University of Mississippi used EEGs to record electrical activity in the brains of three groups of right-handers: gay men, straight men, and straight women. First the researchers recorded electrical activity during a "resting" period to get a baseline reading. Then they recorded while the three groups viewed pairs of words and faces and were asked to judge which one of the pair was happier.

In the baseline recording, the gay group was the *only* group in which one hemisphere of the brain was activated more than the other. In the second recording, the pattern of brain activation in gay men was like straight women's and distinctly different from straight men's. All three groups were equally accurate at judging the emotional content of the words and faces, but it was clear that the women and the gay men were using different parts of the brain than the straight men, suggesting they were employing a different mental strategy to do this task.

It looks as though my initial impression — that the gay men I met through my son actually *thought* differently — may have been pretty close to the mark. As the above findings show, gay men do have their own patterns of cognitive skills and they also have their own patterns of brain activation when they're handling various mental tasks.

OTHER DIFFERENCES BETWEEN GAYS AND STRAIGHTS

A few years ago, researchers in Doreen Kimura's program at the University of Western Ontario decided to compare gay and straight people on physical skills instead of cognitive skills. First they made sure that their subjects didn't differ in hand strength or in experience with sports, which might have given them an unfair advantage in the tests to be used. Then they tested the two groups' skill at throwing a ball and their speed at inserting pegs into a pegboard. In the pegboard test, which measures manual dexterity, both lesbian and straight women were faster than both gay and straight men. On the ball-throwing test, straight men were the most accurate of all the groups but lesbian women were just about as good, and both of them were much better than gay men and straight women. The gay men and lesbians had scored like their own sex in one task and like the opposite sex in the other task. It's obvious then, that in physical skills, as in mental skills, homosexual men and women have their own unique skill sets and cannot be pigeonholed neatly into heterosexual categories.

Body differences between gays and straights have also been reported. A survey of more than 5,000 women found that lesbians on average were taller and heavier than heterosexual women. Social scientists have claimed that these body differences can be explained by factors other than biology. For example, large women may be less attractive to men and therefore more likely to turn to other women as partners; straight women may have weighed less because they were more obsessed with thinness. I'm inclined to disagree with the latter, because the survey data were gathered in the late 1930s to early 1960s, a time when thinness was much less important to most women, as well as to most men, than it is today.

The onset of puberty doesn't differ between lesbians and straight women, but it does between gay and straight men. Gay men on average are younger than straight men at the onset of puberty and also shorter and lighter, a pattern more likely to be found in straight females than in other men.

When researchers find physical differences between straight men and women, they wonder whether those differences might also be present between gays and straights. That's why researchers sometimes compare people on some of the strangest things — inner ear cavities, fingertip patterns, fingertip lengths. Not that any of these things is all that important in itself; it's just that there's an explanation for their difference in men and women (i.e., prenatal hormones), and so perhaps the same explanation may apply to gay and straight people. For example, as reported in Chapter 2, the cochlea (in the inner ear) is more sensitive to soft sounds in women than it is in men. This sex difference is present in infants and children as well as in adults, showing that it's laid down early in development. Armed with this knowledge, neuropsychologists at the University of Texas decided to compare the cochlea of lesbian and bisexual women with those of straight men and women. They found that the cochlea's sensitivity in gay and bisexual females was intermediate between straight females and straight men — less sensitive than in straight women, but more sensitive than in straight men. This showed that the auditory systems of these women had been partially masculinized, probably by prenatal hormones.

It's interesting to note that heterosexual female twins who've shared the womb with a male twin also have the same partial masculinization of the cochlea, implying that the presence of a male in the womb exposed the female twin to an abnormal dose of androgen.

Other researchers examined the auditory systems of gay and bisexual men and discovered that they, like lesbians, were less sensitive than straight women to soft sounds and more like other men. In fact, the auditory systems of these men were "hypermasculine" — that is, even less sensitive to soft sounds than straight men were. Both lesbians and gay men had auditory systems that had been masculinized in the womb.

In 2003, researchers at the University of East London reported yet another neurological difference between straights and gays: the strength of the startle response. The startle response — the way the eye blinks when we hear a sudden loud noise — is controlled by the limbic system, an old part of the brain involved in emotion and in sexual behaviour. The researchers found a huge difference in the strength of the startle response in men and women: men's responses were three times as strong as women's. Both gay men and lesbians were intermediate between straight men and women. The blink response is involuntary; it's "wired in" to the brain from earliest development, and so the finding that straights and gays have different blink responses is yet another indication that sexual orientation is influenced by events in the womb.

Still more evidence of this kind came in 2005 and 2006, when Swedish researchers reported on people's responses to pheromones (chemicals in the brain that evoke a sexual response from another). Gay men and straight women responded to the same pheromones, while straight men and lesbians responded to the same pheromones.

Differences in the pattern of fingertip ridges of gay and straight people have also been reported. You read in Chapter 2 that people who have more ridges on the left hand than the right are in the minority and are usually female. Hall and Kimura discovered that gay men, like women, more frequently have this reversed pattern and, when they do, they're also more likely to be left-handed.

Finger *lengths* too have been shown to vary with sexual orientation. A group of researchers headed by Marc Breedlove and his student Terrance Williams at Berkeley found that lesbians had the more masculine pattern — that is, a shorter index finger than ring finger (measured on the right hand). Most gay men didn't differ from straight men, but the minority of those who did differ showed a "hyper-masculine" pattern — that is, even a greater difference between index and ring fingers than straight men have. An additional finding was that both gay and straight men with two or more older brothers had a more masculine fingertip pattern than men with no older brothers. (Having older sisters made no difference.)

More recently Vindy Brown, Marc Breedlove and colleagues reported that lesbians who identified themselves as "butch" had a more masculine finger-length pattern than lesbians who identified themselves as "femme." The researchers commented that probably the sexual orientation of "butch" lesbians is due to prenatal hormone exposure, while that of "femme" lesbians is not. In 2003, two other researchers tested a group of lesbian twins who were "identical"[†] and found, as expected, that both twins had the more masculine finger-length pattern. They also tested a group of identical twins in which only one of the pair was lesbian, and found that *only* the lesbian twin had the masculine finger length pattern, whereas the straight twin had the typical heterosexual pattern. As these identical twins shared the same genes, their different finger lengths must have been due to differences in their prenatal environment. The second-to-fourth finger length ratio develops during the first trimester of pregnancy, and differs in males and females. The fact that it also

---

† The popular name for monozygotic (MZ) twins, who come from the same egg but are actually not always identical.

differs in straight and gay people reinforces the claim that prenatal hormones are involved in the determination of sexual orientation.

A word of caution regarding the foregoing: don't try to label your friends' sexual orientation on the basis of their finger lengths or number of older brothers. As you know by now, these differences are *averages* including both low and high scores, so they tell nothing about anyone's friends or relations. It's interesting to know these things because of what they may tell us about prenatal hormones or genes, but they're useless for individual diagnosis.

The finding that gay men, at least in some respects, appear to be hypermasculine may seem contradictory to findings that gay men, on some tests, score more like women than like straight men. Nevertheless, gay men do display several hypermasculine characteristics. For one thing, they report having had more sexual partners over their lifespans than straight men, just as straight men report having had more sexual partners than straight women. Also, as you've read in this chapter, gay men have some cognitive skills that differ from straight women's scores more than straight men do. Some gay men also have a hypermasculine finger-length pattern.

Perhaps the most curious finding of all is that, on average, gay men have larger genitalia than straight men. This was first reported in 1961 by Kurt Freund (the plethysmograph researcher mentioned in Chapter 3) and another physician. The finding may be difficult for some straight men to accept, but the same thing was reported in 1999 by Canadian and American psychologists. They analyzed data from more than 5,000 men interviewed by the Kinsey Institute and found that, on average, the homosexual men had penises that were both longer and thicker than those of the heterosexual men. This was despite the fact that the homosexual men, on average, were shorter and weighed less than the heterosexual men. The researchers speculated that differences in penis size could be due to differences in prenatal hormones, caused by genetic differences or differences in prenatal stress. It was known that, in pregnant female rats, prenatal

stress produces an initial surge of testosterone, followed by a permanent decline in testosterone level. If the same is true for humans,
then the early testosterone surge could produce some of the hypermasculine characteristics in gay men (including larger genitalia),
while the later decline in testosterone could account for their more
feminine characteristics.

TRANSSEXUAL BRAINS

Several studies have shown that transsexuals, like homosexuals, have
more non-right-handedness, suggesting that their brains are lateralized differently from others. Even when transsexuals are right-
handed they have a more extreme version of right-handedness, and
that is associated with unusual brain laterality just as left-handedness
is. (Moderate right-handedness seems to be the one associated with
the most typical development.)

When psychiatrist Diane Watson surveyed handedness at the
Vancouver Gender Dysphoria Clinic in 1991, more than 40 percent
of those in the transsexual group proved to be left-handed, compared
to fewer than 12 percent in the control group. Ten years later, in 2001,
a study by Richard Green of the Charing Cross Hospital in England
also reported increased non-right-handedness in transsexuals,
though at a lower rate than reported in the earlier study. Green's
study was huge — more than 500 transsexuals, divided into subgroups according to whether they were asexual or were erotically oriented toward heterosexuals, homosexuals or bisexuals. Regardless of
their erotic orientation, all the transsexual groups had higher rates of
non-right-handedness than the control groups, indicating that they,
like homosexuals, have some brain functions operating differently
from other people.

Earlier you read that a fetus's preference for one hand or the
other has been observed early in gestation. As transsexuals have
unusual handedness, perhaps handedness and transsexualism have a
common origin: both may be due to unusual levels of prenatal

androgen. According to one study, hormones may be a better explanation than genes. That study found that transsexuals were even *more* likely to be non-right-handed if they had no left-handed relatives. (If their non-right-handedness were genetic, they would have more, not fewer, left-handed relatives.)

Transsexuals have also been shown to have anatomical differences in the brain. Dick Swaab and colleagues, who'd been first to report a difference in homosexual brains, reported in 1995 that they'd found a female-sized brain structure in male-to-female transsexuals. Called the *bed nucleus of the stria terminalis* (BSTC), the structure is essential for sexual behaviour. It was already known to be smaller in straight women than men; now it proved also to be smaller in genetically male transsexuals. But couldn't it have been the hormone injections they'd been given to help change their gender to female, that had caused the BSTC to shrink? The researchers checked this out and discounted it. Then, when they examined female-to-male transsexuals, they found that their BSTC was male-sized, just the opposite of that in male-to-females. In other words, transsexuals who felt like women (but were born with a male body) had a female-sized BSTC; those who felt like men (but were born with a female body) had a male-sized one. These findings strongly suggested that transsexuality is biologically determined. The researchers also learned that BSTC size was unrelated to sexual orientation. Whether a transsexual person was attracted to men or to women, the BSTC was the same size.

The Netherlands researchers also found other brain differences in transsexuals. The suprachiasmatic nucleus (SCN) was enlarged in male-to-females, as it was gay men. And the nearby sexually dimorphic nucleus (SDN) was small, as in straight women. Other researchers reported that the corpus callosum in female-to-male transsexuals was more like that of straight males than females.

Taking the above findings together produces the strong impression that in some respects male-to-female transsexuals' brains are like those of straight females, while female-to-male transsexuals' brains are like those of straight males. No wonder these people feel as though they are trapped in the body of the opposite sex!

WHAT ABOUT BRAIN DIFFERENCES *WITHIN* GROUPS?

So far, research on brain differences has looked at *average* differences between one sexual group and another. Of course that doesn't tell us anything about the different sexual shades *within* each group. Straight women who are well above average in masculinity, and straight men who are extremely high on femininity, get lumped in with all the other straight women and men, which would disguise any real differences within each group. The same is true for homosexual populations: masculine and feminine gay men get averaged together under the homosexual label, as do "butch" and "femme" lesbians. But the recent finding that butch and femme lesbians differ in their finger-length pattern (and by implication, their brains) shows that there are indeed differences *within* sexual groups as well as between them. My fond hope is that, as the science of human sexuality continues to grow, future research will address these issues and reveal more about the true breadth and diversity of human sexuality. I fully expect that significant differences will be identified within all of the sexuality groups identified so far.

6

Biology and Sexual Orientation

That is the essence of science: ask an impertinent
question, and you are on the way to a pertinent answer.

JACOB BROWNOWSKI, *The Ascent of Man*

IS BIOLOGY DESTINY?

AS YOU READ through the previous chapters,
you must have noticed several signposts
pointing toward the conclusion that our sex-
ual orientation is rooted in our biology. Some of the evidence is cultural. The fact that homosexuality has been shown to be present in
diverse cultures around the world, including some that are highly
intolerant of it, strongly suggests that it's innate rather than created
by society. So does the experience of boys in New Guinea cultures
(described in Chapter 5) whose years of ritual same-sex behaviour
ought to have made them homosexual if social conditioning were
the cause of it. Instead, almost every one of these boys became a
heterosexual adult.

Then there's the neurological evidence — structural differences between gay and straight brains, differences in how their two cerebral hemispheres are "wired," gay/straight differences in cognitive abilities and handedness. All of these point to a biological cause, and one that occurs very early: it's known that both handedness and brain laterality are laid down early in development. So are the physical differences between gays and straights — different finger lengths, fingertip patterns, penis size — all related to developmental events during gestation.

The *lack* of evidence for family influence on sexual orientation also suggests a biological basis. Several empirical studies have tried to find family causes of homosexuality but failed. The experience of transsexuals is the best argument of all against the notion that the family determines sexual identity and orientation. Despite strong disapproval from family and others, transsexual children and adolescents cling tenaciously to their conviction that they are trapped in the wrong body. So strong is their unhappiness that they are willing to risk alienation from family and others and to undergo lengthy, difficult, painful and costly procedures, sometimes stretching over many years, to make their bodies consistent with their inward feelings.

I don't believe any thoughtful person today can deny that biological events influence our sexual orientation. Instead of asking *whether* there's an influence, the real questions now are *how much* of an influence? And how does it happen? The answers depend on whom you talk to. Biologists, like the rest of us, hold varied beliefs.

Take the sociobiologists, for instance. These scientists, who first became prominent in the mid-1970s, are hardliners, arguing that genes determine everything about us. Richard Dawkins, author of *The Selfish Gene*, describes human beings as "robot vehicles blindly programmed to preserve the selfish molecules known as genes," having no higher purpose in life than to get our genes passed along to the next generation. Biologists like Dawkins, and evolutionary psychologists like Steven Pinker, see a direct causal relationship from our genes to our behaviour and, as the human genome was being mapped out and sequenced, the tendency to attribute more and more of our humanness directly to our genes accelerated. Genes have now been proposed as the basis for a wide variety of human traits and behaviours, including shyness, assertiveness, religiosity, child abuse by stepfathers, depression, criminality and attraction to money and power. It's even been suggested that there may be genes for homelessness! As *The New Yorker* so wisely put it, "biobabble is now driving out psychobabble."

Fortunately, many other scientists reject the "genes are us" school of thought as simplistic and dangerous. They caution that blaming everything on our genes may lead us to abandon our responsibility for changing society's ills. Along with scientists from other disciplines, these biologists argue that, although genes are indeed important, they are not immune from social influences. Of course that goes for sexual orientation, too. If genes are involved in determining sexual orientation, it's unlikely they're going it alone.

THE GENE THEORY OF SEXUAL ORIENTATION

One of the ways of looking for a genetic influence on sexual orientation is to study whether homosexuality runs in twins. The best way to do this would be to study identical[†] twins reared apart in different homes, because then any similarity between them would likely be due to their genes (which they share) than to their home environments (which they don't share). The problem is, separated identical twins are very rare. Researchers have reported that there are only about 200 in the entire world literature.

---

† The terms "identical" and "fraternal" are popular terms for monozygotic (MZ) twins, who develop from one egg and sperm, and dizygotic (DZ) twins, who develop from two eggs and sperms. For convenience, the popular terms are used here without quotation marks, although these terms are not scientifically accurate.

Because of this shortage, researchers do the next best thing: they compare identical twins who've been raised together with fraternal twins who've been raised together. As each set of twins grew up sharing a home environment, any differences between the two pairs should be due to their genes. This way of studying twins has been criticized on the grounds that parents treat identical twins more similarly because they look alike and that treatment, instead of their genes, could explain their similarities in behaviour. However, several studies have shown that this is not the case, at least for the traits studied so far. Identical twins whose parents make an effort to treat them alike do not behave more similarly than identical twins whose parents make an effort to treat them differently.

As noted in the previous chapter, identical twins come from a single fertilized egg, which splits sometime in the first two weeks after conception. Sharing the same egg and sperm, identical twins also share all their genes and therefore they are more alike than other pairs. If homosexuality is genetic, then if one of them is gay, the other one should be, too (at least more often than in other pairs.) Fraternal twins come from two eggs fertilized by two sperm, so they share only about half of their genes and, consequently, are less alike than identical twins. If a fraternal twin is gay, the other one is also likely to be gay more often than ordinary siblings would be.

Why don't identical twins *always* have the same sexual orientation? Because they're not truly identical. Geneticists have observed that identical twin pairs can be different in birth weight, genetic disease and congenital anomalies (for example, if one twin has a congenital brain anomaly, the co-twin typically does not). Identical twins may also differ in their handedness, in the direction of their hair whorls, in the presence or absence of a birthmark and in their risk for contracting HIV from infected mothers. (Differences like these are due to random variations in cell development or to slightly different conditions for each twin in the womb.) In addition, birth factors, including fetal position and the order of delivery, can also reduce the resemblance between identical twins. Thus, even if sexual orientation is genetic, identical twins won't *always* have the same sexual orientation, but they'll have it more often than any other kind of pair because they're still more alike than all others.

So what have we learned from twin studies? Three studies in the early 1990s all found that identical twins were both homosexual more often than were fraternal twins, indicating that a homosexual orientation is highly heritable. Unfortunately, there was a major problem with these studies: they all recruited their subjects via advertisements in gay publications and so the people in these studies were not necessarily representative of the general twin population. Two later twin studies, both using volunteer twins from a twin registry, did not confirm the three earlier studies. However, in the first national study of twins in the U.S., published in 2000 by a group of public health researchers who used scientific sampling instead of volunteers, the results of the three early twin studies were confirmed. This study found that homosexuality occurred in both identical twins significantly more often than it did in fraternal twins and ordinary sibling pairs. Also, in both the fraternal twins and the ordinary sibling pairs, same-sex pairs (more alike than opposite-sex pairs) had the same sexual orientation more often than opposite-sex pairs. There was no evidence that the identical twins' shared childhood environment or adult experiences contributed to their greater similarity for sexual orientation. As in the early twin studies then, these results support the claim that genes are involved in determining homosexuality.

Part of the problem in studying the heritability of sexual orientation is that homosexuality is relatively rare in the general population and therefore, in a small or medium-sized sample of a population, it's difficult for statistical analysis to detect it. In addition, as a Swedish study of breast cancer showed, it can sometimes be very misleading when the scores obtained by people taking part in a study are averaged. Using average scores, the Swedish researchers had found that breast cancer was only moderately heritable. However, later molecular genetic analysis revealed that the study had actually included several different *kinds* of breast cancer, some highly genetic, some moderately genetic, and some very environmental kinds. Lumping together the scores from all these different people had yielded a misleading average.

That last point also applies to other conditions, including hand-edness or sexual orientation. Some left-handedness is due to genes while other left-handedness is due to birth trauma, brain injury or other causes. Some homosexuality may be highly genetic, while other homosexualities may be due to other factors, including environment. If so, then putting these different subtypes together in scientific studies and averaging their scores will conceal or minimize genetic effects that may be there. Studies of sexual orientation need to look at more homogeneous subgroups within a particular orientation. Recent studies comparing highly effeminate homosexuals with other gay men, and comparing "butch" and "femme" lesbians, are a good start.

HOMOSEXUALITY IN FAMILIES

What about other ways of testing the genetic theory of homosexuality? If genes do influence sexual orientation, shouldn't homosexuality run in families? Turns out that it does: all of the modern family studies of homosexuality, stretching over more than two decades, point to a genetic influence on sexual orientation.

One of the most consistent findings in these family studies was a birth-order effect for gay men: they tended to be born significantly later in the family. Being gay was not correlated with having older sisters, younger sisters or younger brothers, nor was it related to the parents' age at the time of a man's birth. The research showed that each additional brother increased the chances of a younger brother being gay by 33 percent, a highly significant increase in odds. (In 2005, a team led by Ray Blanchard reported that the birth-order effect applied only to younger brothers who were right-handed!)

Then other relatives were scrutinized. Dean Hamer reported that gay men had elevated numbers of gay uncles and cousins on the mother's side of the family but not on the father's side, indicating that homosexuality ran in the female line. (Soon gay and lesbian bookstores were selling T-shirts reading *Thanks for the genes, mom.*) On the father's side of the family, Hamer found increased rates of lesbianism and bisexuality in the cousins and nieces, which did not occur in the mother's side of the family. A later study found that, on the father's side of the family, lesbian and bisexual women had elevated numbers of sisters, daughters, nieces and female cousins who were not heterosexual.

Writing in the *Annual Review of Sex Research*, Ray Blanchard of the Clark Institute of Psychiatry in Toronto claimed that "birth order is one of the most reliable epidemiological variables ever identified in the study of male [but not female] sexual orientation." He reported that transsexuals who are gay exhibit the same late birth order as "generic" homosexual groups. Kenneth Zucker and Ray Blanchard later reported that an excess of brothers is usually not seen among samples of homosexuals who were not feminine as boys; it's the most effeminate of gay men who are most likely to have an unusual number of older brothers.

Concerned that research had been limited to white subjects, Anthony Bogaert of Brock University examined data from 823 black men who had been interviewed at the Kinsey Institute for Sex Research from 1938 to 1963. He found that the black gay men had the same late birth order and excess of brothers as had been found for white gay men.

Blanchard and others decided to look for birth-order effects in young boys and male adolescents. These were youngsters who were referred to the Clarke Institute for behavioural treatment of effeminate mannerisms that concerned their parents. Compared to other children and adolescents, these young males proved to have the same late birth order and excess of older brothers as gay men.

Then in 2000, Anthony Bogaert examined the birth order of homosexuals by using the data gathered from the large survey conducted by the Chicago University group in 1994 (described in Chapter 3). As in the previous studies, Bogaert found that gay men were born later in the family than straight men, but there was no such birth order effect for women.

What about lesbians? Though no late birth-order effect has ever been found for lesbians, they do have more gay relatives than other women. In the 1990s Michael Bailey and his colleagues found that 12 to 20 percent of the lesbians they studied had homosexual siblings, compared to only two percent to five percent of the heterosexuals. This finding was later confirmed by other researchers, showing that female homosexuality does run in families. But couldn't lesbians have more lesbian sisters simply because they grew up in the same family? To find out, the researchers compared identical twins, fraternal twins and pairs of adopted sisters. They found that it was genetic closeness, not family influence, that linked to homosexuality. Identical twins were more likely than fraternal twins to both be lesbians, but adopted sisters raised by the same parents were not more likely to become lesbians.

It's clear from the above family studies that a growing body of evidence points to a genetic influence on sexual orientation. Both gay men and lesbians have an increased likelihood of having homosexual siblings. The more older brothers a boy has, the greater his chances of being gay, or gay and effeminate. Gay men also have more gay uncles and cousins on their mother's side of the family and, on their father's side of the family, their cousins and nieces have an increased probability of being lesbian or bisexual. Lesbians have more lesbian siblings and more other non-heterosexual female relatives on their father's side of the family.

The finding of later birth order and more older brothers in male but not female homosexuals has now been reported in many different samples of people in several countries, including the U.S.,

Canada, the U.K. and the Netherlands. If the effect is indeed genetic, questions remain about where the relevant genes might be located, or how they might exert their influence. And what would the relevant genes be doing? It's fairly easy to figure out the role of genes when dealing with simple physical characteristics such as eye or hair color; those traits depend on a gene making a single protein that influences that trait. But for a trait as complex as sexual orientation, the genetic effect would probably come from multiple genes interacting with each other in very complex ways.

It may be a long time before we learn where the relevant gene or genes are, and what they actually do to influence sexual orientation. Perhaps genes make a person more or less sensitive to prenatal hormones, so that one fetus would react strongly and another would be unaffected. Perhaps genes regulate how much of each sex hormone a fetus is exposed to. It's impossible to separate the effects of genes and hormones because each can affect the other. Maybe what genes really do is influence our physical or personality traits, and these in turn influence the social interactions we have that contribute to our sexual orientation. In other words, the true role of genes may be to determine what effect different environments will have on us.

Whatever the (hypothetical) sexual orientation genes do, it seems that those for a homosexual orientation are not dominant. Molecular geneticist Jan Witkowski, who runs the Banbury Center at Cold Springs Harbor Laboratory on Long Island, has been quoted as saying:

If there is a homosexuality gene, it is not dominant ... but it could be recessive, and thus there could be tens of millions of people who are carriers. If you're heterosexual and your husband or wife and your children are heterosexual, that doesn't necessarily mean a thing genetically. If there's a gay gene, one or all of you could be carrying it. Your next child, or perhaps your grandchildren, may by chance get the genetic combination, and suddenly you've got someone gay in your family. (From A *Separate Creation*, by Chandler Burr.)

Genes are tricky players, but despite their prominence these days, it's good to remember that they are not the *only* biological players. As the following sections show, there are several other potential avenues for biology to influence sexual orientation.

THE MATERNAL IMMUNE HYPOTHESIS

I think this is one of the most intriguing theories about the origin of male homosexuality, and possibly the one most amenable to research. The theory is that male fetal tissue may provoke an immune response in the mother, so that she becomes progressively immunized against this tissue with each additional pregnancy. In the 1960s, American biologist Milton Diamond and his colleagues had shown that, in guinea pigs, there existed certain mechanisms that protected the pregnant female from being masculinized by male hormones produced by the male fetus she was carrying. Diamond believes a similar process probably occurs in humans.

This notion has been carried forward by Ray Blanchard and Anthony Bogaert, who speculate that the increased likelihood of a boy being gay when there are older brothers may be due to a maternal immune reaction to only male fetuses. A woman's immune system, having been provoked by a male fetus to produce antibodies, would "remember" the number of male fetuses she has previously carried, and progressively increase its response to the next fetus. That would explain why having older brothers would increase a boy's likelihood of being gay, whereas having older sisters would have no effect, as the mother's immune response is to males only. The hypothesis is based partly on evidence that male fetuses are more antigenic (i.e., more toxic) to the mother and therefore more likely than female fetuses to provoke immune reactions in her. There is already evidence that maternal antibodies to sex hormones are one cause of undescended testes.

The possibility of the mother's immune system "remembering" the number of male fetuses she has carried is supported by a surprising finding by a group of American geneticists and pediatric researchers. They discovered that cells from male fetuses can still be circulating in the mother's blood as long as 27 years after the birth of a male baby, indicating that pregnancy with a male fetus may establish a long-term, low-grade immune response to future male fetuses.

In 2001, Ray Blanchard reported finding that homosexual males with older brothers weighed less at birth than other males. It was already known that this was true for heterosexual males with older brothers; now Blanchard found that gay males with older brothers weighed even less at birth than straight males with older brothers. He found the same things — lower birth weight, more older brothers — in a sample of 250 boys (average age seven) who had been referred for psychiatric treatment because of their cross-gender behaviours. Blanchard conjectures that a mild maternal immune response to male fetuses could produce a slightly reduced birth weight, whereas a stronger immune response could produce an even lower birth weight as well as an increased probability of homosexuality.

The "maternal immune reaction" theory applies only to males, of course. Even if it's true, it doesn't explain homosexuality in females. It also doesn't explain why gay men have not only more older brothers but also more aunts, as Dr. William Turner of the State University of New York reported. Turner looked at more than 200 families who had gay sons or daughters. He found that families with a gay son, but not families with a gay daughter, had twice as many aunts as uncles on the mother's side of the family. The fathers of these gay men did not have the same lopsided ratio of aunts and uncles in their families. Incidentally, this is exactly the case for my own gay sons. They have twice as many aunts as uncles — four to two — on my side of the family but, on my husband's side, they have twice as many uncles as aunts.

What could account for the skewed ratios of aunts and uncles on the mother's side of families with gay sons? Turner proposes a theory of miscarried fetuses (called "fetal wastage"). He calculated that about 35 percent of the males conceived in the mother's family were miscarried, which would produce about 50 percent fewer live male births than live female births. That would explain why there were twice as many aunts as uncles on the mother's side of the family. Turner cites a rather complicated genetic mechanism (which I won't go into here) to explain both the high degree of male fetal wastage in the mother's family and the increased likelihood of the mother's offspring being homosexual.

THE NEUROENDOCRINE THEORY OF SEXUAL ORIENTATION

("Neuro" refers to the nervous system and "endocrine" to the hormone system; hence "neuroendocrine" refers to the influence of hormones on the developing nervous system.)

After reading so much about gay/straight differences in prenatal sex hormones, one might expect that gay men would have lower testosterone levels than straight men. In fact, there is no difference in the amount of testosterone coursing through the bloodstreams of gay and straight men. Several studies have measured that, and all of them came to the same conclusion: whatever differences exist between gays and straights are not due to differences in their adult testosterone levels. That doesn't mean, however, that there were not significant differences in their hormone levels before they were born or soon afterward, which is what the neuroendocrine theory claims.

According to this theory, when prenatal sex hormones from the gonads and the adrenal glands permanently masculinize or feminize the fetus' brain, creating slightly different structural and functional arrangements in the brains of males and females, they also, at the same time, establish a bias in erotic attraction toward one sex or the other.

As you read in Chapter 1, some of the earliest research in this area was on animals. Scientists altered the usual amounts of prenatal sex hormones or changed the timing of exposure to them, and then observed the effect on the animal's subsequent sexual behaviour.

Remember the infant male rats who were castrated and grew up to act like females? And the lambs whose mothers had been implanted with testosterone at different points in gestation and who, when they grew up, showed variations of male or female behaviour, depending on when they'd received the testosterone?

And it wasn't only animals who reacted this way. Remember the human syndromes described in Chapter 1 — all those initials, CAH, AIS, DES? These were people who, for various reasons, had been exposed before birth to sex hormones in unusual amounts or at unusual times. What these syndromes showed was that exposure to too much male hormone in the womb could masculinize human females, while too little of such exposure could feminize human males.

But the hormone story doesn't stop there. Until quite recently, scientists believed that sex hormones were produced only by the testicles and ovaries and by the adrenal glands. Now another surprising source has been discovered: the brain. Sex hormones in the brain are called "neurosteroids" because they're produced within the neurons. In animals they've been shown to affect mating behaviours and also to affect an animal's *response* to mating signals. Researchers at the Institute of Endocrinology in Genoa have postulated that neurosteroids may play a crucial role in forming gender identity in humans. They speculate that androgens may be deficient in the brains of male homosexuals and may also be atypical in the brains of transsexuals, creating a "disconnect" between psychological sex and gonadal sex. If that's true, perhaps neurosteroids also influence all the other shades of human sexuality. Obviously this is a hot area for future research.

DOES PRENATAL STRESS AFFECT SEXUAL ORIENTATION?

This is another proposed contributor to sexual orientation. Studies of female animals who've been stressed during pregnancy (by a variety of procedures, including handling) have reported numerous effects on the offspring. Professor Lee Ellis of Minot State University has done a lot of work in this area. He summarized the effects of prenatal stress to include the following: altered sex differences in cerebral asymmetry and in sensitivity to alcohol; in females, increased male-typical play behaviour and altered parenting behaviour; in males, reduced male mating behaviours and increased female-type behaviours. Apparently what produces these changes are hormones produced by the adrenal glands and released into the pregnant animal's bloodstream when she experiences emotional stress. It's been known for many years that stress hormones in the mother can reach the fetus via the placenta. Once they do, they can depress the production of sex hormones in the fetus and thereby alter the sexing of the brain.

Ellis points out that, in a mature animal, occasional exposure to high levels of stress hormones doesn't appear to have any permanent effects. However, if the exposure to stress hormones occurs at critical periods of an animal's early development, it can cause permanent brain changes, particularly in males, who seem to be more vulnerable. Stress hormones acting on males at critical periods can make the brain less masculine and more feminine.

One study reported that prenatal stress can even affect nerve cells (neurons) in the brain. In the adult offspring of normal rats, the females have longer branch-like dendrites growing out from the ends of their neurons. But in neurons taken from the brains of rats whose mothers had been stressed in pregnancy, the males had longer dendrites. Prenatal stress had reversed the typical sex differences in the brain's neurons.

Does prenatal stress affect human infants, too? Does a pregnant woman's exposure to stress bias her baby's brain toward homosexuality or bisexuality? Some of the earliest studies, in Germany and the U.S., reported that this did appear to be the case, but these results were not confirmed by later studies. One of the more recent studies did find a greater number of effeminate sons of mothers who reported the highest levels of prenatal stress, but the mothers' reports relied on old memories and so they may not have been accurate. Obviously this is yet another area that needs more research.

DEVELOPMENTAL INSTABILITY

In recent years a theory called "developmental instability" has been advanced by psychologists and biologists at the University of New Mexico and the University of Pierre and Marie Curie in Paris. Developmental instability refers to small deviations from the original genetic plan for an organism's development. These tiny departures from the plan are due to "noise" in the system — random variations in the growth and division of cells during development. All of us experience some instability during our development, even if it's only a small amount. Given the list of things that can affect our development, we're bound to run into something — pollution, pathogens, toxins, stress during pregnancy, spontaneous mutations or perhaps "homozygosity" (a genetic term meaning that a person inherits two identical versions of a gene and therefore breeds true for the corresponding characteristic). No wonder nobody's perfect!

Some biologists have claimed that the most sensitive indicators of a person having experienced developmental instability are small deviations from perfect symmetry in the two sides of the body. When the two sides differ in features such as ear levels or fingertip length or the patterns of fingertip ridges, or when the two sides of the brain have unusual patterns of activation when performing cognitive tasks, these things are believed to be products of developmental instability. All of these conditions are more common in left-handers and in people with extreme right-handedness (it's *moderate* right-handers who tend to have the fewest of such conditions.)

In 2000, researchers at Sweden's Karolinska Institute in Stockholm reported the surprising finding that repeated ultrasound exposure in fetal life increased the risk of left-handedness in men, which indicates that prenatal ultrasound affects the fetal brain. The study was very large: almost 7,000 men who had been exposed to ultrasound were compared to 172,000 who were not. Researchers found that, when ultrasound scanning was done at 28 weeks of gestation, there was no increase in left-handedness. However, when a second trimester scan was introduced, along with a second scan at 32 weeks, there was a 30 percent increase in left-handedness. This was attributed to damage to the left or to both hemispheres during the second trimester. If these findings are confirmed in future research, it would be interesting to explore the possible connection between ultrasound and sexual orientation, given the elevated rates of left-handedness in gays and transsexuals.

Martin Lalumiere, Ray Blanchard and Kenneth Zucker at the University of Toronto have concluded that homosexuality is associated with developmental instability. They base this conclusion on the fact that homosexuals, compared to others, have more non-right-handedness, more unusual patterns of brain activation for certain cognitive tasks, less symmetry in finger lengths and in the patterns of fingertip ridges, plus a greater number of older brothers (which Lalumiere earlier showed was related to increased asymmetry). These differences are more common in gay men than in lesbians, which is what one would expect if developmental instability is involved, because girls are much less vulnerable than boys to many developmental problems that are now suspected of being caused by instability in early development of the brain and nervous system. Exactly *how* such disruptive events would modify the brain's erotic orientation is unclear; Lalumiere and his colleagues nominate mechanisms in the hormone and immune systems as candidates. Like many other theories in this field, more research is needed.

BIAS, NOT PREDESTINATION

What you've read in this chapter suggests that a person's sexual orientation begins with an innate bias in the nervous system. Whether the bias toward heterosexuality, bisexuality, homosexuality or transsexuality is determined by genes, prenatal sex hormones, maternal stress, a mother's immune reaction to her male fetus, developmental instability or something else remains to be determined. All of these are suspected influences, and it's possible that each of them may be more influential in some cases than in others.

You may have noticed that I've been careful not to claim that biology *determines* our sexual fate but only that it plays a significant role in it. I've used the word "bias" to describe what I believe happens in the developing nervous system to create the likelihood of a particular outcome. An inborn bias makes one sexual orientation more likely than another, but at times other factors may be strong enough to overrule that bias or at least to reduce its influence.

Moreover, although biological effects are probably strongest in infancy or childhood, they don't end there. They continue as we grow into adulthood and for the rest of our lives, for our bodies and brains are constantly changing in response to our experiences and even in response to our thoughts and changing beliefs. Throughout each day our hormone levels rise or fall; the neurons in our brain grow new branches or lose old ones; our nervous systems replace existing pathways with new ones. In this sense then, the "you" who faces the world each day is not exactly the same "you" who faced it yesterday or the day before. And because you are slightly changed, you will not be affected in exactly the same way by the experiences you encounter tomorrow. The dance between your biology and your external world — your friends, work, family and society — goes on until the day you die.

7

Nature and Nurture— The Dance Goes On

Experience is not what happens to a man; it is what a man does with what happens to him.

ALDOUS HUXLEY, *Texts and Pretext*

THE JULY 17, 2001, *Advocate*, which focused on the theme "Why Are We Gay?" describes a theory by Mark Stoner, who plays the clarinet:

Ever since Stoner, a 41-year-old creative director for an advertising agency in Lancaster, Pa., realized that three out of four of his childhood friends who played the clarinet grew up to be gay, he has taken note of who among his adult gay friends once played the instrument. What he calls an "exhaustive but unscientific" survey covering two decades indicates that "there is an extremely high correlation between playing the clarinet and being gay ... My theory is that most boys want to play the trumpet ... But the more sensitive boys wind up with the clarinet, and we're the ones who turn out gay."

189

Stoner admits he's only kidding, of course, but he's not alone in trying to explain where sexual orientation comes from. Over the past decade or two, several experts, most of whom don't play the clarinet, have proposed a variety of explanations for the origin of sexual orientation. At one extreme are the sociobiologists described in the previous chapter — "biology is destiny"— and at the other end are the social constructionists — "society is all" — described below.

IS SEXUAL ORIENTATION "CONSTRUCTED"?

Social constructionists believe that all of human behaviour, including human sexual identity and orientation, is "constructed" in response to social factors, culture and experience. One well-known spokesperson for this viewpoint is sociologist Pepper Schwartz of the University of Washington, author of several popular books about sex, including *Everything You Know About Love and Sex is Wrong*. In her academic writing, Schwartz denies that erotic desire is an innately fixed quality. Her thesis is that "desire is created by its cultural context. Sexuality emerges from the circumstances and meanings available to individuals; it is a product of socialization, opportunity, and interpretation."

Note that the source of sexuality here is the person's environment and experience rather than a fixed, core, inward sexual desire. Social constructionists speak of homosexual *behaviour* rather than of homosexuality as a fixed trait. Schwartz has argued that we generally tend to think of people "falling in love" and then developing an emotionally intimate relationship, but in women it's often the other way round — desire may be aroused by emotional intimacy rather than by "wired in" erotic taste. A woman meets another woman, says Schwartz, forms a close emotional friendship with her and then finds herself sexually attracted to her. If a woman changes her relationship she can also change her sexual behaviour and her sexual identity. For example, when two heterosexual married women leave their husbands and together embark on a same-sex relationship, they redefine themselves as lesbians.

Social constructionists like Schwartz criticize the biological theory of sexual orientation on several grounds. They point out that the "prenatal hormone" hypothesis is based largely on experiments with animals and they may be affected differently by prenatal sex hormones than humans are. They also reject the evidence from those human syndromes you read about in Chapter 1, in which offspring had received abnormal amounts of prenatal sex hormones. They argue that the increased incidence of homosexuality and bisexuality in these women could be due to social factors rather than to prenatal hormones.

But social constructionists receive their share of criticism, too. The biggest criticism is the lack of empirical data showing *how* society creates different sexualities. Many of the published studies in this area are theoretical and conjectural rather than empirical. Even when social studies do provide empirical evidence for something, the *effect* of that something is often merely assumed rather than proved. For example, social constructionists point to the large number of studies showing that boy and girl infants are treated differently by their parents and others; they infer that this differential treatment of boys and girls is what gives rise to sex differences in behaviour. The problem is that there is no evidence to back up this assumption. It's true that parents do treat male and female children differently, but there is no evidence that that's what causes the difference in the children's play behaviour or, for that matter, in any other behaviour that differs between males and females.

Similarly, Schwartz has cited the English public school as a training ground for homosexuality. "If you want to train boys to be gay," she has said, "send them to an English 'public' school…where their only credible experiences are with their chums." But in fact, research has shown that such same-sex activity in schoolboys does not condition them to become homosexual adults. The 1994 national survey of Britons' sexual attitudes found that, although men who had attended all-boy boarding schools were more likely than other men to report homosexual experience while at school, in adulthood they had no greater incidence of homosexuality than boys who did not attend such schools.

Criticizing the social constructionist view of sexual orientation, psychologists Michael Kauth and Seth Kalichman point out that, instead of social factors creating a homosexual orientation, they actually work against it.

> Americans grow up in an antihomosexual society and in families that do not encourage but rather explicitly and implicitly punish homosexual tendencies. Advertising, music, television, movies, and organized social functions remind us constantly that heterosexual behavior is rewarded, despite moral prohibitions against adolescent or premarital sexuality…. promotion of heterosexuality is loud, clear, and consistent. Within such a society, it seems unlikely that there should be more than occasional same-sex sexual behavior, and people who prefer such activities should be quite rare. [Yet the] prevalence of gay men, lesbians, and bisexuals in western societies suggests that same-sexual behavior is not uncommon.

THE INTERACTIONIST VIEW

Between the two extremes of social constructionism (nurture) and biological essentialism (nature) is the "interactionist" position, which today has many advocates from both the biological sciences and the social sciences. These social scientists concede that biology does contribute to sexual orientation (in some as yet unknown way), but they reject the notion that biological factors directly *determine* it. Most biologists wouldn't disagree with that. Nowadays what usually distinguishes one point of view from the other is the different *emphasis* that each gives to biology and environment in the development of sexuality.

The interactionist model, to which I subscribe, recognizes the important influence of genes and sex hormones on human sexual development but it also notes that the direction of influence can also go the other way: environment and experience can sometimes affect levels of sex hormones and this in turn can affect genes. Although sex hormones can't actually alter the genes themselves, what they *can* do is determine which genes will likely be expressed and which will not.

Geneticists have shown that genes have at least two functions. First, they comprise a stable pattern that can produce exact copies for succeeding generations. This function of the gene is not affected by social experience. But genes also have another function — the ability to code for the production of specific proteins — and this function *can* respond to environmental influence. A person's environment can affect whether, or to what extent, a gene will code for a specific protein, and in this way the environment can determine whether that gene will get fully expressed and affect the person's behavior.

It's been known for a long time now that environment can influence certain physical characteristics such as height. Even though you inherit "tallness" genes from your parents, you may still remain short if you don't receive adequate nutrition while growing up. Japan provided a dramatic example of this. Prior to World War II, most Japanese people tended to be quite short. But after the war the Japanese diet began including more protein, and the increased consumption of protein had the effect of extending the average height of young Japanese by several inches over that of their parents' generation. This was a big surprise to everyone. Before then it had been widely accepted that height was under genetic control: tall people had tall children and short people had short ones. The Japanese experience revealed that environment (in this case, nutrition) could affect the expression of the tallness genes. Without adequate nutrition, these genes were unable to express themselves; with improved nutrition, they were. Of course there were plenty of Japanese people who remained short despite a higher protein intake. These people carried "short" genes instead of "tall" genes, so the new protein environment had little or no effect on them.

But your environment affects more than your genes; it also affects your brain. Information from outside your body is constantly being fed to your brain via the pathways from your senses — sight, hearing, touch, taste and smell. Whenever you have a new experience and learning occurs, changes take place in your brain. Your neurons grow new branches, which form new connections with your other brain cells. Activity may increase in one area of your brain and decrease in another. Existing patterns of connections may be strengthened or weakened. New patterns may be formed to support the new learning you've done. In this way, your brain's activity and even its structure are continually being subtly altered by input received from your environment.

This was illustrated in male mice, in a study of paternal behaviour. If a baby mouse inches away from the nest, adult males who've never had contact with baby mice won't retrieve the wandering baby. However, put the adult males in the company of baby mice for a few hours and they then *will* retrieve the wanderers. What changed? The researchers examined the brains of the changed mice and discovered that spending time with the babies had actually altered the activity of the estrogen receptors in their brains, making their behaviour more paternal.

Although adult brains can change, experience during early life may produce the biggest changes because the brain is developing most rapidly at that time of life. It's now widely accepted that the basic ground plan for the brain is laid out in our chromosomes, but the precise details of the brain are determined by our experience, including our experience in the womb. A baby is born with about 50 trillion neurons in its brain, but neurons can only become functional in response to stimulation from outside, primarily from parents. Early in life, the neurons in an infant's brain that are stimulated the most form networks for processing information, while other neurons die off.

Even apparently "natural" processes such as learning to see or to speak cannot develop without environmental stimulation. A baby would never learn to see if its eyes were covered and unable to receive stimulation from outside itself. And it would not learn to talk if it didn't hear language spoken by its parents and others. In the normal course of events, of course, infants do receive the required stimulation and are able to learn both seeing and talking.

The rare occasions in which infants did not receive adequate human interaction have provided dramatic examples of the effect on the nervous system. Biologist Anne Fausto-Sterling, author of *Sexing the Body*, describes what happened to two children in India early in the 20th century, when they were raised from infancy by a pack of wolves. "The two girls could run faster on all four limbs than other humans could on two. They were profoundly nocturnal, craved raw meat and carrion, and could communicate so well with growling dogs at feeding time that the dogs allowed the girls to eat from the same bowls. Clearly these children's bodies — from their skeletal structure to their nervous systems — had been profoundly changed by growing up with nonhuman animals."

As babies grow to adulthood, an array of influences — from the social environment, from the individual's own behaviour and from changes in the individual's hormone levels — can all produce changes in the brain. Experiments with rats showed that those raised in an "enriched environment" that included rat toys and varied activities ended up with a thicker cortex in the brain than rats raised alone in a non-enriched environment. On the other hand, rats raised in a stressful environment grew up to be much more reactive to stress in adulthood. This was true even for rats who'd been bred to handle stress well. A bad environment could overcome their genetic predisposition not to become stressed.

Elderly brains too can be changed by their environment. Years ago, research by neuroscientist Marian Diamond showed that elderly rats, whose brains were comparable to those of a 90-year-old human, grew new branches on their neurons when new challenges were introduced into their environment. More recently, neuroscientist Marc Breedlove showed that raising the testosterone levels of adult female rats to the same level as males would, within weeks, increase the size of one region in their brain to that of normal males.

Breedlove also showed that the connection also works in reverse, from behaviour to brain. Specifically, he demonstrated that the frequency of sex can alter the brain's neurons. Compared to celibate male rats, sexually active male rats had smaller nerve cells in the areas of their spinal cord that are involved in erections and copulations. Extending the implications of this to humans, Breedlove speculated that differences in human sexual behaviour may *cause* some of the observed differences in brain structure, rather than being caused by them.

I think studies such as these show how fruitless it is to continue debating whether nature or nurture is the root of our behaviour. The two are so intertwined that only an interactionist model of human behaviour makes sense. Any particular behaviour may be more or less the result of your nature or of the nurture you receive, but there is no longer any doubt that both play a role in everything about you. As psychiatrist Dr. Daniel Siegel says in *The Developing Mind*:

> Genes and experience interact in such a way that certain biological tendencies can create characteristic experiences. For example, certain temperaments may produce characteristic parental responses. These responses in turn shape the way in which [the child's] neuronal growth, interconnections, and pruning (dying back) occur ... The question isn't "Is it heredity or experience?" but "How do heredity *and* experience interact in the development of an individual?"

Writing about sex differences, June Reinisch and Stephanie Sanders of the Kinsey Institute in Indiana describe a "multiplier effect" (E.O. Wilson's term), which could just as easily apply to differences in sexual orientation as to differences between men and women:

> Small sex differences in appearance, behavior, and responsiveness at birth combine with cultural expectations about appropriate behavior for each sex and lead to augmentation of the behavioral sex differences. Each successive interaction alters the organism slightly. The modified organism then perceives and responds to the environment a little differently and, in turn, is perceived and treated in a slightly different fashion. Through this dynamic transaction between the organism and its environment involving biological, psychological, and social factors, major sex differences in behavior emerge over time.

Reinisch and Sanders explain how biology interacts with culture. "The prenatal hormonal environment may affect behavior by biasing the neural system in such a way as to create behavioral predispositions. It is then that culture adds its influence by rewarding, punishing and/or ignoring behaviors and thereby can exaggerate, diminish, distort or permit the expression of biologically based ... differences."

Environmental factors — stress, social experience, physical illness — can affect whether our genes will have a large or a small impact on us. For example, susceptibility to psychotic illnesses is genetic, but whether the relevant genes have a large or a small impact can sometimes depend on what's happening in the person's life. With some physical illnesses, the person's psychological condition determines whether the illness ever develops, even though the person carries the genetic marker for that illness. For example, one study compared a group of people who carried the marker for rheumatoid arthritis but did not develop the disease, to another group who carried the marker and did develop the disease. The only feature distinguishing the unaffected group from the affected group was the former's good psychological health, which managed to inhibit the expression of the genetic marker for the disease.

Steven Rose, author and director of the Brain and Behavioural Research Group at Britain's Open University, writes eloquently about how organisms are "active players in their own destiny," shaped by their environments but at the same time choosing, shaping, or creating those environments. He describes the continuous interchange between us and our environment, which he calls the "interdependence" of our genes and our experience. Rose eschews the kind of "simplistic, reductionistic" thinking that attributes human characteristics directly to genes. He emphasizes that the expression of a gene depends on the environment within which it operates. Some environments may encourage its expression while other environments will discourage it.

In addition, the same environment can affect people differently because we all experience the environment through our own genetic "filters." For example, let's imagine there are genes for homosexuality and two brothers both inherit those genes. Rose would say they'd be more likely to develop that orientation if they grew up in a family that was more tolerant of that orientation and *also* if, biologically, they had a temperament that was highly responsive to their environment. In those circumstances, one brother, whose temperament was well attuned to his environment, might develop the homosexuality encoded in his genes, while the other brother, with a temperament that made him resistant to the influences of his environment, might not develop that orientation even though he had the same predisposing genes for it and the same tolerant family environment.

A person's *beliefs* can also affect whether or not an inborn predisposition for something ever gets expressed. Beth Casey and her colleagues at Boston College showed that having a biological predisposition to develop masculine characteristics never got played out in girls who perceived that their parents would disapprove. It was only when girls perceived that their parents would approve of masculine characteristics that these actually developed.

But the direction of influence between biology and environment can also go the other way: biological factors, if strong enough, can make one immune to social influence. Sociologist J.R. Udry studied daughters who had received low or high levels of testosterone in the womb (as measured in their mothers' amniotic fluid, which had been frozen). He found that the low-testosterone girls were more easily influenced by their mothers. When mothers encouraged typical femininity, the daughters tended to be feminine; when mothers encouraged typical masculinity, the daughters tended to be masculine. But the high-testosterone girls were generally masculine in their behaviour, regardless of their mothers' expectations and encouragement. The high level of prenatal testosterone they'd experienced in the womb was strong enough to make them immune to their mothers' later social influence.

Steven Rose writes of developmental "plasticity" — the ability to adapt to our environmental demands and to compensate for deficiencies. But he points out a big *but*, and this is important: plasticity is limited; it can only occur within the range set by the genes. That's why the same environment can have different effects on different individuals: each of us has individual genetic limits. As the Japanese experience showed, increased consumption of protein enabled the tallness genes to be fully expressed in people with "tallness" genes but not in those with "shortness" genes. Even so, there was a limit to how tall people could grow; their height couldn't exceed the upper limit set by their genes. This is also true of personality characteristics. A friendly environment may help a shy person to become less shy, but it cannot turn him into an extrovert.

In my psychology practice I sometimes had a patient whose brother or sister would become my patient some years later, for an unrelated matter. I was always impressed by how one person's genetic limits had caused her to experience her parents and her family environment so differently from her sister with different genetic limits. When each of these siblings described their parents and recalled their family environment, it often sounded as though the parents were two different sets of people and the home two different places. It wasn't that one patient had a better memory than the other; it was simply that each had experienced her family through her own genetic filter. Consequently, each had formed a different set of beliefs about the family.

But it's not only our genetic limits that cause us to be differently affected by the same experience. It also depends just *when* a particular event occurs. If it occurs at a critical period in our development, it may not be susceptible to later social influence. Sexologist John Money points out that when nature and nurture interact at a critical period in prenatal or postnatal life, the programming that occurs may be irreversible. On the other hand, if the same programming occurs in a non-critical period, it may be much more malleable. Animal studies showed that a good social environment could overcome a rat's failure to mate properly if the rat's problem was caused by social stress, but the good environment had no effect if the problem was caused by exposure to insufficient androgen in early life. The lack of androgen at a critical period had limited the rat's developmental "plasticity" — its potential to benefit from later corrective intervention.

Different personality traits are also affected differently by our genes. Twin studies have shown that how much genes and environment each contribute depends on which trait is being measured. For example, genes shape individual differences in personality, such as extroversion or introversion, to a greater degree than they shape individual differences in traits such as work satisfaction. Also, as Nancy Segal points out in *Entwined Lives*, genetic influence on a trait doesn't mean that it's totally resistant to change. For example, children born with phenylketonuria (PKU), a genetic metabolic error that causes mental retardation, can still be treated early with special diets that largely offset this mental effect.

INTERACTIONS AMONG GENES, HORMONES AND ENVIRONMENT

In my opinion, the bulk of the evidence so far suggests that human sexual orientation results from complex interactions among our genes, our sex hormones and our experience. In her book, *Sexing the Brain*, Australian neuroscientist Lesley Rogers describes observing these interactions in her work with chicks. She notes that chicks' brains are lateralized: the left hemisphere is specialized for learning to recognize food, the right hemisphere is specialized for controlling sexual and aggressive behaviour. Dr. Rogers demonstrated that the chick's brain gets lateralized as the result of interactions among genes, sex hormones and environment.

Just before hatching, almost all chick embryos are oriented inside the egg with a leftward twist of the body (that's *genetic*). Because the body is twisted leftward, it blocks the embryo's left eye from exposure to light entering the shell; only the right eye is exposed to light (that's the *environment*). The light promotes the development of more connections between the right eye and the brain than between the left eye and the brain, so that each cerebral hemisphere ends up being specialized differently. But this difference between the hemispheres is greater in males than females because they each receive different exposures to prenatal sex hormones (the *hormone* effect), and that hormone exposure interacts with the light before hatching. (In contrast, both male and female chicks that are not exposed to light until *after* hatching do not develop lateralized brains.)

How complicated development is, even in chicks! Imagine then how much more complicated human development must be, with immensely more complex interactions among our genes, our sex hormones and our environments. We may accept the interactionist model as a general picture of how sexuality develops, but even so, we are still a long way from understanding its specifics.

WHICH ENVIRONMENT?

What do we mean when we say "the environment" interacts with our biology? Which environment? The home? The school? The church? The workplace? The people we hang out with? All of these? Until fairly recently, when social scientists spoke of the influence of "nurture," they were referring to the home environment in which a person was raised. They assumed that parents were the ones who would have the most influence on their children's personality. The problem is, parents provide the child's genes and also the child's environment, so it was impossible to distinguish the effects of one from the effects of the other.

The ideal way to study this would be to study identical twins reared apart in different homes. Identical twins are genetically more alike than any other human pair and therefore, when they're reared apart, differences in their personalities should be due primarily to their different home environments. But as you read in the last chapter, there are too few separated identical twins in the world to make such research practical. Instead, researchers study unseparated twins and other kinds of relatives to untangle the effects of genes and environment. They compare identical twins with fraternal twins and with non-twin siblings. They measure the effects of home by comparing the similarity of siblings from the same home to the similarity of siblings raised in different homes. They measure the effects of genes by seeing how much adopted children differ from the other siblings in the home. They also compare adopted children to both their biological siblings and their adoptive siblings.

In *The Nurture Assumption*, Judith Rich Harris summarizes the results of this research. For most psychological characteristics, heredity accounts for about 50 percent of the variation among people; environmental influences account for the other 50 percent. (Harris notes that most of the populations studied so far have been American and European, and mostly middle class, so these percentages may not apply to other populations.)

The 50-50 split between nature and nurture is probably no big surprise to anybody. It's pretty obvious to most people that genes and environment are both important players in human development. But, as Harris reports, another more recent finding by these researchers was a huge surprise: they discovered that the most influential environmental factors for shaping adult personality were those that were *not shared* by siblings. In other words, it is not your family environment, the one you and your siblings shared as you grew up, that has the major influence on how your genes get expressed. It's the environment *outside* the family, the experiences that are unique for you and for each of your siblings, that makes the difference.

Many people, including social scientists, parents and adult children, find this difficult if not impossible to accept. Surely parents must be the greatest influence on shaping their children's personalities! What about those studies we learned about in Psych 101 showing that criminals raise criminals, abusers raise abusers, responsible parents raise responsible children? Harris says she subscribed to all of these views during her lengthy career of writing developmental psychology textbooks, until she discovered that none of these studies had controlled for heritability (genes). Instead of trying to prove causation, all these studies simply implied that *correlation* meant *causation*, that is, if two things occur together, it can be assumed that one caused the other — a common error in research. Responsible parents do tend to have responsible children, but that doesn't mean that the parents' responsible behaviour *caused* the kids' responsible behaviour. It could just as easily have been the genes they share that made them both responsible people.

Harris notes that, if parents were the primary agents for molding their children's personalities and behaviour, then the adopted children and stepchildren they raise should also be like them. But in fact, as the newer studies were showing, adopted children and stepchildren are not like the stepparents and adoptive parents who raised them. Moreover, these studies also showed that, when biological parents and kids were similar, their similarities were more likely to be due to their shared genes than to their shared home environment. The studies also showed that almost all the similarities between adult siblings can be attributed to their shared genes, instead of to growing up in the same home.

Harris also notes that identical twins reared in the same home are no more alike than identical twins who were separated as infants and raised in different homes. Isn't that surprising? It's hard to believe that twins wouldn't be less alike if they grew up in different homes but, according to the research Harris cites, none of us was greatly affected by the family home. (The exception is families that are *seriously* dysfunctional; these families *do* affect the children's adult personalities.)

But if it isn't generally the influence of the parental home that affects us most, what *does* (besides our genes)? According to the findings of behavioural geneticists, our most influential environment is the one we *don't* share with our siblings — that is, the experiences we have outside the home that are unique for each one of us. Foremost among these influences, according to Harris, are other kids. She argues (and a lot of research backs her up) that, although a close attachment to mother or mother substitute is essential for the healthy development of babies and toddlers, the socialization of older children is done mostly by the children's playgroup.

Obviously this is too huge and contentious a topic to pursue further in this book, but anybody who wants to know more can read

Harris' book. Whether you agree with her or not, the book is a fascinating read. I cite it here principally to draw your attention to the possibility that the home environment you think of when you talk about "nurture" interacting with "nature" may in fact not be the relevant environment at all. Instead, it may well be the friends you grew up with, the things you (and none of your siblings) did with others outside the family, that affected you most.

So what has all this got to do with sexuality? Just this: the finding that family environment is not the major contributor to personality and behaviour fits well with other researchers' findings (cited earlier) that no family variables were strongly implicated in the development of sexual orientation. Perhaps sexual orientation, like other characteristics, is shaped by the family's unshared experience. Some authors have suggested that the relevant environment for playing out a biological bias for sexual orientation is the individual's peer relationships in the years preceding and following puberty. Sounds plausible to me, but empirical studies are needed to see whether in fact it's true.

TWO "INDIRECT" MODELS OF SEXUAL ORIENTATION

The "interactionist" model of human sexual orientation, in which biological factors interact with environment to produce a certain orientation, is probably the most widely accepted model these days, and various versions of it have been proposed. Here are two of the most interesting:

New York psychiatrist William Byne believes that biological factors don't directly determine sexual orientation, but they do shape a person's temperament and other personality traits, and those in turn influence how that person interacts with his environment, how he interprets events and experiences them internally. For one person, biology will play the major role in determining sexual orientation, whereas for another person it would play only a minor role.

Byne gives the example of a boy who tends to avoid the competitive rough-and-tumble play typical for young boys, a tendency that's known to be influenced by prenatal hormones. (These boys have been shown to have an increased likelihood of being homosexual in adulthood.) A direct biological model of sexual orientation would say that the boy avoided typical boy-type activities because in the womb his brain received less androgen, which "wired" it both for avoiding rough-and-tumble play and also for adult homosexuality. Byne's indirect model would say that what biology determined was the boy's temperament and it was *that* which led him to avoid typical boy-type activities. In turn, avoiding typical boyish activities would become a potent factor predisposing the boy to homosexual development, but *only in certain environments*. For example, he might be raised in a home that labeled him a "sissy" because he avoided competitive boy-type play or, alternatively, in a home that fully accepted his "unboyish" behaviour and encouraged him to choose girls instead of boys as playmates if he did not enjoy playing with boys.

Psychologist Daryl Bem of Cornell University has proposed another indirect model of sexual orientation. Like Byne, Bem suggests that genes code for childhood temperament, and temperament influences the child's preference for playmates and play activities. But Bem's model has an interesting twist. In this model, preferring "unboyish" friends and activities would make a boy feel different from other boys, and he would come to view their differentness as "dissimilar from me, unfamiliar, exotic, romantic." Thinking these thoughts, the boy would experience heightened arousal of his autonomic nervous system, creating a feeling of excitement when he viewed other boys. This feeling would subsequently get eroticized, as explained below. In Bem's words, the "exotic becomes erotic." On the other hand, close childhood familiarity with the opposite sex would either extinguish erotic/romantic attraction for that sex or prevent it from developing in the first place.

That last sentence reminds me of a former patient of mine. She was born on a farm in a remote area of the Canadian prairies. Her only playmates were her three older brothers, whose games she learned to play "like one of the boys." Hoping to encourage more "girlish" behaviour, her mother bought her a doll buggy for her sixth birthday. Mysteriously, the doll buggy went missing soon afterward. It was eventually discovered, stuffed behind the furnace in the basement. It was never played with. The girl grew up showing no interest in clothes, makeup, cooking or any of the other "female" interests in which her mother tried to involve her. She became a very good athlete. After high school she dated boys a couple of times, but didn't feel romantically inclined toward them. Soon afterward, she formed a sexual liaison with a young woman from her basketball team. When I met her, she had been involved in another lesbian relationship for many years. In Bem's model, this woman's close childhood familiarity exclusively with males (her brothers) had prevented her from feeling erotic attraction to males in adulthood.

In support of his theory, Bem points out that virtually all human societies polarize the sexes to some extent, "superimposing a male-female dichotomy on virtually every aspect of communal life. These gender-polarizing practices ensure that most boys and girls will grow up seeing the other sex as dissimilar, unfamiliar, and exotic — and, hence, erotic." But how does exotic get turned into erotic? By exciting the autonomic nervous system, says Bem, and associating that inner feeling of excitement with the object that caused the arousal. Bem cites the well-documented observation that novelty and unfamiliarity produce heightened arousal in humans, and argues that the novelty of the same sex — a novelty caused by that sex not being available in childhood — could produce the same autonomic nervous system arousal that other novelties produce. Bem also cites extensive experimental evidence that an individual who has been physiologically aroused by a target will show heightened sexual responsiveness to it. In this case, the "target" would be members of the same sex, to whom one had been physiologically aroused because of their novelty.

Bem's notion that the child's choice of playmates indirectly determines his sexual orientation is consistent with Judith Rich Harris's report that children are primarily socialized by their peer group. As most children play and do things with kids of the same sex after early childhood, most children would grow up to be heterosexual. The minority of children who prefer opposite-sex playmates and activities would grow up to be homosexual. Thus, in this scheme, the "gene for homosexuality" would actually be a gene (or genes) for a temperament that leads to atypical childhood activities and playmates, and that's what sets off the chain of behaviours leading to homosexuality.

THE DANCE GOES ON

Whatever the genes do, and whatever the relative contributions of biology and social experience may be, it seems clear that both play their part in the development of our sexuality. The particular complement of genes you received created your unique "genetic limits," which cause you to experience your environment in particular ways and to draw your own personal meanings from your experience. How you act upon your environments, and are in turn affected by them, depends partly on what kind of a person you are. What tendencies have already been built into your nervous system, your hormone system, your immune system? These tendencies encourage you to interact in certain ways with your parents, your siblings, your friends and co-workers, and to feed back to your brain the meanings that you alone can draw from these interactions.

But your biological constraints do not rob you of free will. I reject firmly the notion that we are genetic pawns in the game of life, but I just as firmly reject the notion that we can become anything we want to be. Our genes set limits, and change that's induced by our environment can only take place within those limits. Biology defines the range within which each of us must operate and determines how influential the environment can be on each of us. Apart from transsexuals, men cannot become women, nor women men, regardless of their environment. Society may encourage men and women to become more androgynous, to blur their differences in terms of clothing, work and other activities, but that will not change their sexual identity. Similarly, homosexuals and heterosexuals cannot change places, regardless of their environment. They may imitate one another's behaviour, and sometimes do, but that doesn't alter their basic erotic orientation.

Although all of us are influenced by both our biology and our life experience, for some people biology probably plays the major part, whereas for others, society is the more influential. Remember, though, just because an influence is social doesn't mean that it's changeable, particularly if it occurs at a critical point in development. John Money calls this "developmental determinism." "Whether the determining agents of homosexuality (and heterosexuality) are innate and biological or acquired and social is beside the point. The point is that they are determinants, no matter where they come from, or when they occur." Some social experiences can permanently alter the nervous system, just as biology can.

8

If It's Normal,
Why All the Fuss?

We can be absolutely certain only about things we do
not understand.

ERIC HOFFER, *The True Believer*

INTOLERANCE — PRIVATE AND PUBLIC

IVEN WHAT WE now know about sexual
orientation, it seems absurd to think of it
as a wilful choice, just as it would be
absurd to think of skin colour or left-handedness as choices. While I
was writing this chapter, several new scientific studies were published, all strongly supporting the view that hormonal conditions in
the womb lay the foundation for future sexual orientation. There is
also new evidence that trying to "cure" homosexuality can cause not
only shame, but suicide. And a recent book, *Evolution's Rainbow* by
Joan Roughgarden of Stanford University, catalogues sexual diversity
throughout the entire animal kingdom, including humans, and
argues that such diversity is normal and evolutionarily advantageous.

Nonetheless, many people persist in seeing members of sexual minorities as abnormal misfits. Consequently, the suicide rate for gay teens still remains much higher than that for straight teens. The rate of suicide attempts in gay and bisexual adolescents ranges from 20 to 39 percent, compared to 1.5 to 4 percent in non-gay adolescents. In my own city of Vancouver, a Grade 9 student climbed upon a ledge on the Pattulo Bridge one chilly day in March and jumped. In a suicide note he told his parents he could no longer handle the daily bullying and homophobic insults at his school.

Research has shown that when young people are exposed to low levels of victimization such as occasional name-calling, supportive families can help them cope, but if the victimization is more extreme, families are totally helpless to protect the mental health of their gay children. Many gay teens, unable to find acceptance at school or at home, take to the streets as male prostitutes. The Badgley Committee, which studies child sexual abuse and child prostitution in Canada, discovered that a large majority of juvenile male prostitutes are gay. Once on the streets, their risk of contracting HIV is higher than that of female prostitutes. Studies of street youth in Toronto and Montreal found that, of the youths who tested positive for HIV, almost all were boy prostitutes.

As for adult homosexuals, death by "gay-bashing" still rivals death by suicide. In Vancouver not long ago, a 41-year-old gay man was brutally murdered in Stanley Park by a group of young men wielding baseball bats and pool cues. At an outdoor memorial for the victim, one speaker quoted from a local survey of gay men the previous year in which 45 percent of those surveyed reported that they had experienced physical violence at some point in their lives. So common was such violence, apparently, that most people had never bothered to report it to the police. It was painfully obvious to the assembled crowd that, although gays and lesbians in Canada had made great strides in enshrining human rights in law, too many of their fellow citizens still harboured strong and sometimes dangerous ill feelings toward them. The situation is the same in many other countries, where both official and private discrimination are still all too common.

Prejudice against homosexuality has a very long history. In his book *Homophobia: A History*, Byne Fone describes how homosexuality was first defined as a sin and then later as a crime. The first recorded executions of homosexuals took place in Ghent in 1292. In Florence in the last half of the 15th century, 15,000 men were tried for sodomy crimes; 2,000 were convicted. Fone documents the varied punishments of homosexuals, which included solitary confinement, life imprisonment, banishment, flogging, castration, being exposed in the pillory and stoned, drowning, burial alive, burning at the stake, garrotting, beheading, hanging, being thrown to the dogs and being disembowelled with a hot poker.

Only in the last half of the 20th century did many countries begin legalizing sexual relations between men. Britain retained the death penalty for sodomy until 1861, when it was replaced by life imprisonment. Not until 1986 were all laws against sodomy between consenting adults in Britain repealed.

In the U.S., sodomy statutes remained on the books in 17 states until 2003, with penalties ranging up to life imprisonment (Idaho). Lesbians and gays in the military are still subject to discharge if they reveal their sexual orientation. The official policy is "Don't Ask, Don't Tell," but ex-President Clinton admitted the failure of the military to implement this policy in a fair way. The Servicemembers Legal Defense Network reports that over 10,000 men and women have been discharged from the military for being gay under "Don't Ask, Don't Tell." Even federally funded religious charities are allowed to discriminate in employment, on the basis of sexual orientation.

Such official attitudes are in line with the private attitudes of most Americans. In Gallup and Roper polls over the years, and in questionnaires completed by university students, a majority of respondents have reported that they would not like to work with a gay person or have one for a neighbour. In a 2003 *New York Times-*

CBS poll, 49 percent of Americans answered No to the question "Do you think homosexual relations should be legal?" as compared to 41 percent who answered yes. (In the southern U.S., the proportions were 59 to 32 percent.) Even in states where it's against the law to discriminate against homosexuals in housing, jobs or services, discrimination occurs anyway. Both verbal and physical assaults on lesbian and gay women and men are *the most common kinds of bias-related violence in the U.S.* The horrendous image of young Matthew Sheppard, who in 1998 was tied to a fence in Wyoming and pistol-whipped to death, shocked the entire world. One of Sheppard's murderers, Aaron McKinney, testified, "Being a verry [sic] drunk homophobik [sic] I flipped out and began to pistol whip the fag with my gun." As one observer noted, McKinney offered his hatred of homosexuals as an excuse, as though it were similar to drunkenness in being a mitigating factor in the attack.

In Canada homosexuality was a federal crime until 1969, and it was not until 1978 that homosexuals were accepted as immigrants. In a June 2001 *Maclean's* article, Sue Ferguson reported that gays and lesbians in the Canadian military were once targeted as "the enemy within." She described the "Security Panel" that operated between 1959 and 1968 (at the height of the Cold War). The Panel targeted the Royal Canadian Mounted Police (RCMP), the military and the public service, investigating 9,000 men and women suspected of homosexuality. About 400 people lost their jobs. As Ferguson writes, "The RCMP formed a 'character weakness' unit ... to scrutinize civil servants' backgrounds for evidence of alcoholism, extramarital affairs or anything else that might make them vulnerable to blackmail. Within a few short years ... character weakness had become a code word for homosexual, and sexual practices became the primary area of investigation." To help root out undesirables, a psychologist designed a bizarre device akin to a lie detector for identifying homosexuals. Fortunately, the device, dubbed "the fruit machine," did not work. Although tolerance gradually increased (as civil service unions grew stronger, notes Ferguson), policies prohibiting the employment of gays and lesbians in the RCMP continued until 1988, and it was not until 1992 that the Canadian military officially ended its discriminatory policies against homosexuals.

ARE GAY-BASHERS SECRETLY GAY?

It's long been suspected that men who are homophobic are actually suppressing their own homosexual desires. Are brutal acts by police and some other males driven by their suppressed sexual feelings for other men? Many people have claimed this, but there was no empirical proof to back up such assertions. Then in 1996 psychologist Henry Adams and colleagues at the University of Georgia investigated erotic arousal in a group of straight men, who admitted, on a homophobia index, that they had negative feelings toward homosexuals. The researchers compared these homophobic men to a group of non-homophobic men. Both groups were shown sexually explicit videotapes of heterosexuals, lesbians and gays, while their penile arousal was measured by a plethysmograph. The results? Both groups of men were sexually aroused by videos of both straight and lesbian women, but *only* the homophobic men became aroused by male homosexual videos.

It looked as though these men, who professed to reject homosexuals, actually themselves harboured sexual feelings for other men. To rule out the possibility that the arousal might have been produced by feelings of aggression incited in the homophobic men when they viewed sexy videos of gay men, researchers also administered an aggression questionnaire to both groups. There was no difference in the two groups' aggression scores, which ruled out aggression as the cause of sexual arousal in the homophobic men. Were these men unconscious of their erotic arousal by other men, or were they conscious of it but concealing it, perhaps even from themselves? The researchers were unable to say. My own guess is that some homophobes may indeed be unconscious of their motives while others are fully conscious of their erotic arousal but are bolstering their struggle to repress it by attacking it in others.

Who is likeliest nowadays to feel negative about sexual minorities? Research has consistently shown that people with limited education and people harbouring authoritarian attitudes and traditional ideas about proper roles for men and women are those most prone to hostility toward gays and lesbians. So too are people who are religiously conservative. But the most important factor of all is *never having known a gay man or woman*. This is especially true of straight men. People, especially men, who have never known gays personally are much likelier to subscribe to popular myths about them. Here are three of the biggies:

THE MYTH THAT "MAJORITY MEANS NORMAL"

This is based on the belief that large numbers are superior to small ones: "If the majority of people are a certain way, then obviously that must be the right way to be; why else would most people be like that?" The next step, inevitably, is to brand those who aren't in the majority as abnormal: "Isn't it obvious? If this were a normal guy like me and practically everybody else, he'd be cruising chicks instead of other deviates."

Curiously, it rarely occurs to people who reason thus to apply the same logic to handedness: "Practically everybody's right-handed, so left-handers must be abnormal, disgusting. Let's force them to be normal." Most Western people, of course, no longer hold this view of left-handers, whereas disapproval of homosexuality is still thriving.

THE MYTH THAT HOMOSEXUALS ARE SICK AND THE MYTH THAT HOMOSEXUALITY IS JUST A PREFERENCE

These two myths are closely related because both assume that homosexuals could change their orientation if they wanted to, either by getting "cured" or by simply switching their sexual "preference" to heterosexual. People who believe the "sickness" myth don't view homosexuals as freaks; they regard them as mentally disordered, needing psychiatric help to enable them to recover from their illness and join with normal society. And, in fact, until 1973 the psychiatrists' bible, the *Diagnostic and Statistical Manual of Mental Disorders* (DSM), did list homosexuality as a mental disorder. Once gays and lesbians began coming out of the closet in sizeable numbers, however, psychiatrists were forced to back down. Led by Dr. Robert Spitzer of Columbia University, the 1973 convention of The American Psychiatric Association (APA) struck the offending section from the manual. Its inclusion in the first place had been completely unscientific: there had been no controlled studies showing that gays and lesbians were mentally disordered. The offending section in the DSM was replaced with a diagnosis of *ego-dystonic homosexuality*, a state whereby homosexuals were unhappy about being gay. In 1988, that section too was dropped.

STEREOTYPES

Closely related to myths about homosexuality are various popular stereotypes of gays and lesbians that have repeatedly been reinforced through mass media, schoolyard bullying and religious bigotry. Here are some of the most common stereotypes that have been described by social scientists:

1   *Gay men and lesbians are not "real" men and women.* Lesbians are seen to be undermining the status of the family and of the "real women" in society. Gay men are believed to be effeminate and unmanly, a state that can be very threatening to straight men who need the security of feeling macho. Such men see effeminacy as "letting down the side," undermining the masculinity of the entire male sex.

2   *Gay men and lesbians choose to be "outsiders," refusing to conform to the norms of decent society.* Gay men are seen to flaunt their

sexuality, be flagrantly promiscuous, and evade "normal" responsibilities of family and children. (Sociologists have noted that outsiders — gays, blacks, immigrants, Jews — have often been perceived as threatening the dominant group, particularly in societies that highly value conformity.)

3   *Most lesbians wish they were men.* At the same time, lesbians are stereotyped as man-haters and competitors (with straight men) for other women.

4   *Gay men are pedophiles.* This is the most vicious stereotype of all. Pedophilia has nothing to do with homosexuality. The vast majority of pedophiles, in fact, are straight men who are, or were, married. Nonetheless, many people still believe that gays and lesbians should not be allowed around children. The Boy Scouts of America were embroiled for a decade in a lawsuit brought by Scout leader James Dale when he was expelled from the Scouts after twelve years in scouting. (In Canada and most European countries, boys of any sexual orientation can be Scouts.) Many parents supported the U.S. Scouts' no-gay policy on the basis that gay Scout leaders might encourage their sons to become gay. In response, Steven Cozza, a (straight) young Scout campaigning to allow gays in the Scouts, quipped, "I went to a Catholic School and I didn't become a nun." In August 1999, New Jersey ruled in Dale's favor. The court battle had lasted eight years, and Dale was jubilant. But his joy was short-lived. The scouting organization appealed the case to the Supreme Court, which in June 2000 voted 5-4 against Dale, ruling that forcing the Scouts to accept a homosexual leader placed an unconstitutional burden on the organization's "expressed purpose."

Although all of the beliefs about sexual minorities described above are false, their influence is widespread, even among younger people. In surveys of straight American university students, men generally held more negative attitudes toward homosexuality, but women who scored high on "authoritarianism" also tended to be very homophobic. These were women who modelled their opinions on those of authority figures they respected, especially religious authority figures. Both male and female students were more negative about potential contact with a gay person of their own sex than with a gay person of the opposite sex.

"CURING" HOMOSEXUALITY

At the 2001 convention of the American Psychiatric Association, Dr. Robert Spitzer surprised everyone when he presented a then-unpublished study arguing that "highly motivated" homosexuals may be able to convert to heterosexuality. Part of the surprise was due to the fact that Spitzer had been instrumental in having homosexuality removed from the APA's list of mental illnesses in 1973. Moreover, the APA had denounced supposed cures for homosexuality in 1994. Now Spitzer was claiming that homosexuals could be "cured," which implied that it was an illness. An avalanche of criticism followed, centering on Spitzer's questionable methodology. He had telephoned 143 men and 57 women who had sought help to change their sexual orientation, and asked them if their heterosexual experiences were satisfying. On the basis of their responses, Spitzer had concluded that 66 percent of the men and 44 percent of the women had achieved "good heterosexual functioning." But the answers were purely subjective, unsupported by any external validation such as physiological arousal to heterosexual erotic pictures. Also, some of those who had "changed" had received help from religious groups who were strongly opposed to homosexuality, so those seeking help may well have been persuaded to give up their homosexual behaviour without changing their underlying orientation. Another study presented at the same APA meeting reported that, of 202 homosexuals who tried to change, 178 failed to do so.

A friend of mine from university days tried very hard to overcome his homosexual orientation. A bright, talented guy, Don (not his real name) paid his way through the UBC Social Work program by play-ing piano in a bar. Following graduation he headed for California because he'd heard of a psychiatrist in Los Angeles who "cured" homosexuality. After four years of treatment, Don married a divorced woman 10 years older than he and the mother of four school-age children. If the psychiatrist then wrote "cured" in his case notes, he was sadly mistaken. Don tried desperately to be a good husband and father, but his sexual longing for other men never left him. He stayed with his wife for 15 years, leaving only after the children were grown. Back home in Canada, Don finally allowed himself to live as a gay man. He continued his career in social work and said he was truly content for the first time in his life. Tragically, his life ended when he was murdered in a gruesome hate crime.

In a review of "conversion therapy" for homosexuals published in a public policy text, Douglas C. Haldeman, a counselling psy-chologist in Seattle, notes that efforts to cure homosexuals seem to be increasing nowadays, especially from "pastoral care providers" (church members who purport to give spiritual guidance). Not only is there the question of professional ethics in trying to cure some-thing that is not a mental disease and that is extremely important to an individual's identity, says Haldeman, but there is also the question of efficacy: do conversion therapies actually work? Haldeman's answer is a resounding *no*: "... not only are conversion therapies unethical and professionally irresponsible ... but they additionally constitute inadequate and questionable science." Also, "... these interventions do not shift sexual orientation at all. Rather, they instruct or coerce heterosexual activity in a minority of subjects, which is not the same as reversing sexual orientation."

Haldeman reviews some of the early behavioural treatments for homosexuality, which included giving electric shock or nausea-induc-ing drugs while the subject viewed same-sex erotic pictures: "... such methods applied to anyone else might be called by another name: torture. Individuals undergoing such treatments do not emerge heterosexually inclined; rather, they become shamed, conflicted, and fearful about their homosexual feelings."

As for the religion-based conversion programs, Haldeman says that many of them promise "change" but privately acknowledge that celibacy is actually the realistic goal for homosexuals. (Can you imagine a so-called treatment program asking heterosexuals to permanently avoid sex?) Most of these programs are operated by people without professional credentials who answer to no professional regulatory body. Haldeman notes:

> The fundamentalist Christian approaches to conversion treatments have been characterized by a host of problems, ranging from lack of empirical support to the sexually predatory behaviour of some counselors ... To exacerbate the potential harm done to naïve, shame-ridden counselees, many of these programs operate under the formidable auspices of the Christian church, and outside the jurisdiction of any professional organization that might impose ethical standards of practice and accountability on them.

The lack of success of conversion therapies argues against both the notion that homosexuality is a sickness that can be cured and the notion that homosexuality is merely a preference. In 1990, the American Psychological Association stated that scientific evidence does not show that conversion therapy works and, moreover, that it can do more harm than good. The American Psychiatric Association followed suit in 1994 by denouncing supposed cures for homosexuality. In 2002, the American Psychological Association passed a resolution on "Appropriate Therapeutic Responses to Sexual Orientation." Commenting on this resolution, Dr. Gregory Herek said, "Attempts to use psychological interventions to change sexual orientation are based on the claim that homosexuality is a disease ... [which is] an attempt to use the language of science to promote antigay prejudice. That view is completely inconsistent with the bulk of scientific research and the official policies of the American Psychological Association and the American Psychiatric Association." Attempting to persuade a gay man to become straight is rather like asking a black person to become white.

RELIGIOUS OPPOSITION

In 2003, after months of bitter infighting, the Episcopal Church U.S.A. confirmed the election of its first openly gay bishop when senior bishops voted 62-43 to approve the election of the Rev. Gene Robinson of Minneapolis. The election set off an immediate uproar in the international Anglican Church, particularly in the developing world, which had already been shocked by the Anglican Church of Canada's support for blessing same-sex unions. The Canadian church signalled that it was prepared to walk away from its international church body but agreed to defer the issue of same-sex blessings until the meeting of its general synod in 2007.

Meanwhile, the Vatican, which had earlier issued a strong denunciation of gay marriage, announced its intent to prevent homosexuals from becoming priests. It also launched an inspection of Roman Catholic seminaries in the U.S. to look for "evidence of homosexuality" among existing priests and to root out faculty members who "dissent from church teachings." Not all Catholic priests were happy with the Vatican's stance. In 2006, in an unusual public dissent with their leaders, nineteen Quebec priests published an open letter taking issue with the Church's opposition to both same-sex marriage and the ordination of active gays into the priesthood. "In these matters," said the letter, "the official teaching of the Church has shown itself more than once to be wrong." Writing in *Time*, Andrew Sullivan, who is Catholic, pointed out that the Church's new direction made it increasingly difficult, if not impossible, to "breathe the love of God as a gay Catholic." In the past, noted Sullivan, all that mattered so far as sexual orientation was concerned, was that a priest remain celibate; it was not *who he was* that mattered, it was *what he did.* Now the new Pope had identified a group of people who, "regardless of how they behave or what they do, are beneath serving God."

Religious objection to homosexuality is often based on opposition to non-procreative sex or to any desire that draws men away from their duty to mate with women. Jesus never spoke of homosexuality, but the Bible made it clear that the purpose of marriage was the procreation of children. If a couple had been married 10 years without producing offspring, that was deemed sufficient reason for divorce. Polygamy was not forbidden in the Bible and in fact is mentioned frequently without condemnation. Presumably polygamy was approved of because made it easier for people to follow the biblical injunction to "be fruitful and multiply."

Joan Roughgarden reports that, in the Hebrew Bible, eunuchs were originally banned from the temple, but later the prophet Isaiah clarified that eunuchs were indeed welcome there if they honoured the Sabbath. Roughgarden also points out that both Jesus and the Apostle Philip reached out to eunuchs: In Matthew 19:11-12, Jesus acknowledges the multiple types of eunuchs — the intersexed, the castrated and the self-castrated — and says that the kingdom of heaven is open to them all if they will receive his message. The Apostle Philip actually baptized a eunuch (who also happened to be black) and welcomed him into the Christian church. This welcoming of eunuchs, says Roughgarden, ended when the Christian church substituted celibacy for castration, and monasticism became the new Christian masculine ideal.

Sometimes the religious objection to homosexuality is based on certain texts, such as the following biblical passages:

Thou shalt not lie with mankind, as with womankind: it is abomination.

Leviticus 18:22

If a man also lie with mankind, as he lieth with a woman, both of them have committed an abomination: they shall surely be put to death; their blood shall be upon them.

Leviticus 20:13

Be not deceived: neither fornicators, nor idolaters, nor adulterers, nor effeminate, nor abusers of themselves with mankind ... shall inherit the kingdom of God.

I Corinthians 6:9

For this cause God gave them up into vile affections: for even their women did change their natural use into that which is against nature: And likewise also the men, leaving the natural use of the woman, burned in their lust one toward another, men with men working that which is unseemly ...

Romans 1:26–27

The first passage above was cited by Dr. Laura Schlessinger, an American radio talk show host who dispenses advice to people calling in to her syndicated show, despite the fact that her Ph.D. is not in psychology but in a physical field. Dr. Schlessinger told her listeners that, as an Orthodox Jew, she believed homosexuality was an abomination that couldn't be condoned.

In response to Dr. Laura's citing the passage from Leviticus, Kent Ashcraft, a musician in Bowie, Maryland, wrote her a letter. When she failed to reply, Mr. Ashcraft's friend posted the letter on the internet as "An Open Letter to Dr. Laura":

Dear Dr. Laura:
Thank you for doing so much to educate people regarding God's law. I have learned a great deal from your show, and I try to share that knowledge with as many people as I can. When someone tries to defend the homosexual lifestyle, for example, I simply

remind them that Leviticus 18:22 clearly states it to be an abomination. End of debate. I do need some advice from you, however,
regarding some of the specific laws and how to best follow them.

When I burn a bull on the altar as a sacrifice, I know it creates
a pleasing odor for the Lord (Lev.1:9). The problem is my neigh-
bors. They claim the odor is not pleasing to them. How should I
deal with this?

I would like to sell my daughter into slavery, as it suggests in
Exodus 21:7. In this day and age, what do you think would be a
fair price for her?

I know that I am allowed no contact with a woman while she
is in her period of menstrual uncleanliness (Lev.15:19-24). The
problem is, how do I tell? I have tried asking, but most women
take offense.

Lev. 25:44 states that I may buy slaves from the nations that are
around us. A friend of mine claims that this applies to Mexicans but
not to Canadians. Can you clarify? Why can't I own Canadians?

I have a neighbor who insists on working on the Sabbath.
Exodus 35:2 clearly states he should be put to death. Am I morally
obligated to kill him myself?

A friend of mine feels that even though eating shellfish is an
abomination (Lev.11:10), it is a lesser abomination than homosexuality. I don't agree. Can you settle this?

Lev. 21:20 states that I may not approach the altar of God if
I have a defect in my sight. I have to admit that I wear reading
glasses. Does my vision have to be 20/20, or is there some wiggle
room here?

I know you have studied these things extensively, so I am confident you can help. Thank you again for reminding us that God's
word is eternal and unchanging.

Since the "Dear Dr. Laura" letter was published, Dr. Laura has
broken with Orthodox Judaism, to which she had converted seven

years earlier. She told her radio audience of some eight million listeners that she had received loving and supportive faxes from Christians but no support from her Jewish listeners. Critics have observed that Dr. Laura knows which side her bread's buttered on — the fundamentalist Christian side. (In 2000, the Canadian Standards Broadcast Council warned of complaints that the program was "abusively discriminating vis-à-vis gays and lesbians." Very few radio stations in Canada now carry the program.)

Dr. Laura's critics are not alone in noting how the Bible can be used to justify discrimination. In an editorial in the *British Journal of Sexual Medicine*, Paul Woolly wrote:

> The Church of England no longer supports doctrines such as that espoused in 1 Corinthians 14:35 ("It is a disgraceful thing for a women to speak in church") and accepts that society is radically different today. Women are ordained as priests in the Church of England ... Some modern theologians will point to these inconsistencies and ask the question: "How can traditionalists condone a change in Scriptural doctrine with regard to women, but continue to keep such doctrine with regard to homosexual men?" Others will point to the Church's relative silence on other moral issues, such as sex outside marriage and adultery. According to Scripture, all are sexually immoral acts and equally sinful.

The majority of Christians and Jews nowadays agree with Dr. Woolly that society has changed radically since biblical times. They therefore ignore outmoded biblical injunctions. But many conservative religionists still cite anachronistic biblical or Koranic teachings to justify their opposition to equal legal rights for homosexuals. Even Supreme Court Justices in the U.S. have sometimes cited biblical teachings when they uphold the constitutionality of statutes that discriminate against gays. And when statutes banning discrimination do manage to get passed, religious institutions are often exempted from them.

Clearly, religious opposition is a major stumbling block in the attainment of equal rights for sexual minorities in the U.S. and elsewhere.

Yet many American churches actively support sexual minorities. The Religious Institute on Sexual Morality, Justice and Healing was formed in 2001, apparently as a counterbalance to the religious right. The Institute recognizes sexuality as central to a person's humanity. It promotes a sexual ethic "focused on personal relationship and social justice rather than particular sexual acts," which is code for inclusion of gays and lesbians. The Institute's Declaration is a "consensus statement created by theologians and ethicists from a broad range of religious traditions and currently endorsed by over 2200 religious leaders across the United States, including denominational leaders, seminary presidents, deans, faculty members, and clergy from more than 35 religious traditions." So far the Institute has provided speeches and workshops for dozens of national, state and local groups. It has also presented sessions at various seminaries and divinity schools and offered training workshops to staff at corporations, universities, congregations and institutions across the country. It has developed an "Action Letter" for religious leaders and an "Open Letter to Religious Leaders About Sex Education," which is a theological affirmation of comprehensive sexuality education. It has also worked with the media to help reporters understand sexuality and religious issues. Unfortunately, the Institute isn't nearly so well-funded as are the many groups operating within the American religious right.

THE WINDS OF CHANGE

Despite most of what you've read in this chapter so far, the outlook for improved tolerance of sexual minorities is probably better than it's ever been, at least in Western countries. Elsewhere, improvement is slow or non-existent. As recently as 2000, China officially denied that it had any homosexual citizens, but in the following year (under pressure from Western psychiatric organizations), it removed homosexuality from its official register of psychiatric disorders. Chinese psychiatrists continue to describe homosexual acts as "abnormal," however, and any public display of homosexuality still carries the risk of immediate detention for "disturbing social order."

Most African and Islamic countries too are hold-outs. In 1999, the President of Uganda heard a rumour about a gay wedding and ordered the arrest of all homosexuals. In 2003, a heterosexual Ugandan lawyer, Sylvia Tamale, was voted the worst woman of the year by *New Vision*, a government-owned newspaper, after she lobbied the country's equality commission on behalf of homosexuals.

In Iran in 2005, two teenage boys were publicly hanged for having a homosexual relationship. Homosexual acts are also punishable by death in Afghanistan, Pakistan, Saudi Arabia, Mauritania, Sudan and Yemen. In her book *Nine Parts of Desire*, journalist Geraldine Brooks describes the punishments set down for homosexual sodomy in present-day Iran: "If the partners are married men, they may be burned to death or thrown to their deaths from a height. If they are unmarried, the sodomized partner ... is executed, the sodomizer lashed a hundred times. (The variation in the penalty reflects the Muslim loathing of the idea of a man taking the feminine role of the penetrated partner). Lesbian sex, if the women are single, draws a hundred lashes. Married lesbians may be stoned."

Contrasting with these very conservative views are the changing views in many other countries. As a review article in *The Economist* pointed out, the direction of change is unmistakable almost everywhere except in the Islamic world. The article noted that, in places such as Japan, Brazil and Turkey (a secular country with a Muslim majority), where homosexuality has traditionally been regarded as abnormal and distasteful, the first tentative signs have begun to appear. Homosexuals in these countries are slowly emerging from the closet, sometimes living openly instead of being forced into marriage, initiating small gay pride parades, beginning to publish gay stories and poetry, opening the first gay resort. As governments have become democratic — as in Eastern Europe, South Africa and Spain —

reported *The Economist*, repressive legislation against homosexuality has been replaced by decriminalization and sometimes by prohibitions against discrimination.

LEGAL RIGHTS FOR SEXUAL MINORITIES IN THE U.S.

In the United States, although tolerance of sexual minorities still lags behind that in most other Western countries, progress has been made in several areas. In 1996, the U.S. Supreme Court ruled that homosexuals could not be singled out for official discrimination merely because of hostility or prejudice toward their sexual orientation. This was the first time the highest court in the land had treated gay rights as a matter of civil rights. Since then, public official attitudes toward gays and lesbians in the U.S. have gradually improved in several areas.

In 2000, Vermont became the first U.S. state to legalize civil unions. The same year, the U.S. Court of Appeals ruled that police officers in a small Pennsylvania town had violated the constitutional right to privacy of a local high school football player, when they threatened to "out" him to his family and others. (The youth, Marcus Wayman, had committed suicide just hours after the threat.)

In June 2000, the U.S. Senate voted to include sexual orientation as one of the categories to be covered by a proposed federal hate-crimes bill. Three months later the House of Representatives went on record for the first time as being in support of including sexual orientation in the bill. (Strong opposition from Republicans in Congress, however, prevented the bill from becoming legislation.)

But the biggest breakthrough for sexual minority rights in the U.S. came on June 30, 2003, when the U.S. Supreme Court considered a case brought by two gay men who had been arrested after police, acting on a false report of a crazed gunman, had entered the apartment of one of the men and found the two engaged in sex. Their lawyer argued successfully that the state's sodomy law (which banned both oral or anal same-sex genital contact) violated their constitutional right to privacy and their right to be treated the same as heterosexuals. The Court voted 6 to 3 to strike down all state sodomy laws, which were still on the books in 13 states. In doing so, the Court ruled that consenting adults have a right to engage in private homosexual conduct. This was a complete turnaround for the Court, which 17 years earlier had ruled that the constitution's mention of "liberty" did not cover the right to engage in what society considers "deviant" acts. In making that earlier ruling, which upheld the law in 24 states where homosexual behavior was criminal at the time, the Court had cited the "ancient roots" (meaning biblical) of proscriptions against homosexuality. After the 2003 ruling, Lambda Legal Defense lawyer Ruth Harlow was quoted as saying, "This is an historic day," alluding to the fact that this new law was made on grounds that contradicted biblical teachings.

Another victory for the gay rights movement came in 2004, when the Republican-controlled House of Representatives emphatically defeated a proposed constitutional amendment to ban gay marriage (backed by President Bush but previously rejected by the Senate).

Massachusetts legalized same-sex marriage in 2004, but in 2006, the state's Supreme Court ruled that gay couples living in other states where gay marriage was prohibited couldn't marry in Massachusetts. Eleven states banned gay marriage through public referenda in 2004; since then, numerous other states have followed suit. Legal challenges to these bans have been mounted in several states, but opponents of gay marriage, funded by the religious right, have been on a judicial winning streak. At the time of this writing, only Massachusetts and New Jersey permitted gay marriage, and only Vermont and Connecticut permitted civil unions for homosexual couples.

Meanwhile, conservative writer and television guest David Brooks of the New York Times has been publicly advocating gay marriage. Pointing out that nearly half of all marriages in the U.S. now end in divorce, Brooks writes: "Marriage is in crisis ... Faced with this crisis, we conservatives [should] do everything in our power to move as many people as possible ... to the path of fidelity." Brooks claims that the proper conservative course is not to banish gay people from making marital commitments, but to *expect* them to make such commitments. "We shouldn't just allow gay marriage. We should insist on gay marriage," writes Brooks. "We should regard it as scandalous that two people could claim to love each other and not want to sanctify their love with marriage and fidelity."

Brooks's concern was based on the current demographic of American households. According to U.S. Census data, fewer than one-third of America's households mirror the traditional view of the family — a couple living with their children. How many of those couples are legally married is not reported, but an earlier census reported that married couples living together with their children comprised only 25 percent of American households. Even so, the U.S. public is obviously not ready to bolster those numbers by adding gay couples to the marriage roster.

Most Americans still condemn homosexuals as immoral and feel uneasiness or downright hostility toward them. This is painfully obvious in the biennial National Elections Study conducted by the University of Michigan's Center for Political Studies. Part of the study is a "feeling thermometer battery" that asks respondents to rate their feelings toward groups or individuals in American society. Since 1984, when gays and lesbians were first included in the feeling thermometer battery, Americans have consistently identified them as the most despised and least liked social group in the U.S. (Over the years, however, the proportion of respondents rating homosexuals at o has declined). A *Newsweek* poll conducted in 1992 found that 45 percent of Americans considered gay rights "a threat to the American family and its values," and following the U.S. Supreme Court sodomy decision, public support for same-sex unions plummeted. A Gallup poll conducted in July 2003 found that 57 percent of Americans would oppose a law allowing homosexual couples to form civil unions, up from 49 percent two months earlier. The number of Americans who said they supported same-sex unions dropped from 49 to 40 percent during the same period. When a *New York Times*-CBC poll asked Americans, "Do you think homosexual relations should be legal?" 49 percent said no, compared to only 41 percent who answered yes. (In the southern U.S., as mentioned earlier in this chapter, the proportions were 59 versus 32 percent). Forty-four percent of respondents believed homosexuality to be a choice, while the same number believed it was something a person couldn't change. The pollsters said that the anti-gay views reflected in the poll were the strongest since the question was first asked in 1992.

It's obvious that the issue of gay marriage has spurred a strong backlash in the U.S., where religious affiliation and social conservatism are both higher than in other Western countries. Currently, there are some 45 well-funded religious organizations crusading against gay marriage in the U.S. Their stated agenda is to stop same-sex marriage through the courts. At the forefront of these groups is Liberty Counsel, headquartered in Longwood, Florida. Its president and general counsel, Mathew D. Staver, told a *New York Times* correspondent, "We will use every means the law can provide. This is the central command center for the defense of traditional marriage against the same-sex marriage movement." One of the several victories enjoyed by Mr. Staver's firm so far was a restraining order to stop the mayor of New Paltz, New York, from issuing marriage licenses to same-sex couples.

As for gay adoption, laws vary from state to state. In many cases, one partner adopts a child and then the second applies to become a co-parent. At the time of this writing, California, Massachusetts, New Jersey, New Mexico, New York, Ohio, Vermont, Washington, Wisconsin and Washington, D.C., allow adoption by openly gay and lesbian couples, while Florida is the only state with an outright ban on gay adoption. In Mississippi, a single person may adopt but not a same-sex couple. In Utah and New Hampshire, no unmarried couples, gay or straight, may adopt.

The violent backlash against gay marriage (and increasingly, against gay adoption) is at variance with a track record among Americans since the early 1990s of supporting legal rights for homosexuals, despite feeling little personal affection for them. A majority of Americans support having gays in the military. The Pentagon, after the Persian Gulf War and again after September 11, 2001, suspended discharge proceedings against soldiers who admitted they were gay. Joan Roughgarden, author of *Evolution's Rainbow*, observed that "apparently gay and lesbian troops were just fine in time of war."

Dozens of states, counties, cities and towns in the U.S. have now established some type of benefit or recognition for domestic partners of gays and lesbians and have passed laws penalizing crimes motivated by hatred for homosexuals. Numerous government departments and agencies have adopted non-discrimination policies that include sexual orientation.

In addition, many private employers are taking action on their own. Wal-Mart, the world's largest retailer, has added "sexual orientation" to its anti-discrimination policy and runs a diversity-awareness training program for employees. Motorola, Shell Oil, American Express, First Union and many other large financial services companies first began providing health and other partner benefits to unmarried employees, and, for the first time in 2005-2006, the State of the Workplace report showed that a majority of Fortune 500 companies were offering domestic partner health insurance benefits. In addition, 86 percent of these companies included sexual orientation in their non-discrimination policies and 81 percent included gender identity and/or expression, marking a tenfold increase from 2001.

Some employers are going beyond same-sex partner benefits by pushing the concept of their workplaces as "welcoming places." The Minneapolis offices of American Express, which began offering domestic partner benefits to same-sex couples in 1997, now also requires its employees to go through a Safe Place training program to learn ways of fostering inclusivity at work, such as showing zero tolerance for anti-gay comments or jokes.

At the same time, religious conservatives are working hard to roll back such benefits. The Gay Rights Information website reports numerous actions in American universities, schools, companies and corporations that are contrary to the interests of gays and lesbians:

- AirTran Airways in Orlando fired a gay flight attendant for kissing his boyfriend.
- The Air Transport Association, based in Washington, D.C., sued the city of San Francisco because of its pro-gay domestic partners law.
- The American Red Cross bans even HIV-negative homosexuals from giving blood.
- Barnes & Noble, Inc. pulled the magazine *POZ* off the shelves of some locations after pressure from anti-gay conservatives.
- Baylor University in Waco, Texas, has a policy of expelling students who reveal that they are gay.
- Big Brothers/Big Sisters in the Owensboro, Kentucky, chapter bars homosexual volunteers.
- Bishop Gorman High School in Las Vegas fired a teacher after he mentioned in his personal website that he was gay.
- Bob Jones University in South Carolina bans homosexual alumni from campus.
- Brigham Young University in Hawaii successfully lobbied the Hawaii legislature to exclude from its housing non-discrimination bill any housing owned or leased by religious organizations.
- Brown County United Way in Indiana removed "sexual orientation" from its non-discrimination policy to accommodate the Boy Scouts of America.
- The *Buffalo Jewish Review* refused to run an ad featuring the Buffalo Gay Mens' Chorus because it "might influence young people to experiment with a sexual lifestyle that could be harmful to their health," said the editor.

- The *Caledonian-Record* in Vermont has a policy of not publishing same-sex civil union announcements (even though these unions are legal in Vermont).
- The *Charlotte Observer* in North Carolina refused to put a photo in the paper that showed two men with their faces close together, as though intending to kiss.
- Clear Channel Communications, Inc. in San Antonio, Texas, took down a billboard ad for a gay dating and news site, following complaints from an anti-gay marriage group in Massachusetts.
- *The Columbus Dispatch* in Columbus, Ohio, bans gays from advertising in their main personal ads page. It also publishes the names of homosexuals arrested for having or seeking consensual sex.
- DaimlerChrysler Corp. pulled advertising from an ABC network TV show *Ellen* because of its lesbian themes.
- *Dateline NBC* joined with the anti-gay website Perverted-Justice.com to set up gay males seeking other males online for consensual sex. *Dateline* used hidden cameras to record the men's meeting and expose them on TV.
- Delta Air Lines, based in Atlanta, reprimanded a gay man who kissed his boyfriend on a flight, had the man detained by authorities in Rome, and denied access to his return flight and to future Delta flights forever.
- Denny's Restaurant in Turlock, California, had a lesbian couple forcibly removed because they kissed and sat "too close" together.
- ExxonMobil Corp., after merging with another company, ended its same-sex domestic partner benefits and rescinded Mobil's policy banning anti-gay bias.
- Federal Express Corp. sued San Francisco because of its pro-gay domestic partners law.
- The *Gainesville Times* in Georgia stopped printing a gay newspaper when anti-gay groups requested it to do so.
- Hardee's Restaurant in Johnson City, Tennessee, enacted a "no earrings on males" policy to fire men suspected of being gay.

- The Illinois Railway Museum forced its president to resign after she acknowledged that she was transgendered.
- J. C. Penney Company, Inc. pulled advertising from the TV show *Ellen* because of its lesbian themes.
- KARK Television in Little Rock, Arkansas, KAMR in Amarillo, Texas, KBTV in Beaumont, Texas, WSMN in Nashville, WTVA in Tupelo, Mississippi, and WTWO in Terre Haute, Indiana, all refused to carry the gay-themed program *The Book of Daniel* after receiving pressure from an anti-gay group.
- KETV and KHGI in Nebraska refused to run pro-gay ads against a statewide same-sex marriage ban, but did run anti-gay ads *for* the initiative.
- The *Maine Sunday Telegram* refuses to run announcements of same-sex commitment ceremonies, even though the paper's editor himself was involved in such a ceremony.
- Mariner Mall in Superior, Wisconsin, will no longer host a local youth fair because the fair now includes a support group for gay teens.
- Northwest Airlines, Inc. of Minneapolis refused to allow a gay couple to use tickets that one of them, an employee of the airline, won at a company party.
- The *San Luis Obispo Gazette* and *San Luis Obispo Magazine* will not allow the paper and magazine to portray homosexuals in a positive light.
- Sullivan University in Kentucky told a transgendered student that she had to use a separate washroom because women students objected to her using theirs.
- The Tufts-New England Medical Center in Boston denied a gay man's request to freeze his sperm in its sperm bank because they believed it put them at risk of contracting HIV.
- *Tulsa World* in Oklahoma refuses to allow the word "lesbian" in its newspaper ads.
- The United States Olympic Committee threatened to sue organizers of the Gay Olympics for trademark and/or copyright

infringement, forcing them to change the name to "The Gay Games." (Similar threats were not made to the "Para-Olympics," the "Special Olympics" or the "International Police Olympics.")

- The United Way of Forsyth County, North Carolina, removed anti-discrimination based on sexual orientation from its partnership agreements so as not to conflict with the anti-gay stance of the Boy Scouts of America.
- The United Way of Northeast Florida increased funding of a Boy Scout chapter in the area in case the Scouts' gay ban might be hurting them financially.
- The University of the Cumberlands in Williamsburg, Kentucky, expelled an openly gay student after he came out on a website.
- The University of North Dakota attempted to fire an openly gay choir director.
- The University of Notre Dame in Indiana bans acceptance of advertisements from lesbian and gay alumni in the *Notre Dame Observer*.
- *The Washington Post* published the names, occupations and addresses of men arrested for allegedly engaging in consensual sex at Conway Robinson Memorial State Forest in Gainesville, Virginia.
- Wendy's Restaurant pulled advertising from the TV show *Ellen* because of its lesbian themes.
- West Town Mall in Madison, Wisconsin, would not permit same-sex couples to take part in a Valentine's Day Kiss Off Contest, which was limited to heterosexuals.
- All of the following TV stations aired on their news programs a secretly taped videotape of homosexual men having consensual sex: KENS in San Antonio; KGTV in San Diego; KOMO in Seattle; KPRC in Houston; WCAU in Philadelphia; and WTVR in Richmond, Virginia.

LEGAL RIGHTS FOR SEXUAL MINORITIES IN CANADA

Reform has been much easier to implement in Canada than in the U.S., in part because Canada has a federal Criminal Code that applies in all Canadian provinces and territories. A single modification of that Code in 1969 was sufficient to decriminalize sexual activity between same-sex persons everywhere in Canada. In the U.S, however, most law that discriminates against gays and lesbians is the responsibility of the individual states and cities, and so the struggle for gay rights there has to be waged on a state-by-state, city-by-city basis.

The first major reform in Canada was removing homosexuality from the Criminal Code. Declaring in 1967 that there was "no place for the State in the bedrooms of the nation," Justice Minister (later Prime Minister) Pierre Trudeau initiated an overhaul of those sections of the Code dealing with sexual behaviour, marriage and divorce. In 1977, Quebec became the first province in Canada to pass a gay civil rights law making it illegal to discriminate against gays in housing, public accommodation and employment. The following year, Canada's Immigration Act was amended to admit homosexual immigrants.

It was the federal Charter of Rights and Freedoms, enacted in 1982 and guaranteeing equality to all Canadians, that gave a huge push toward equal treatment of sexual minorities. Numerous successful legal arguments based on the Charter have now secured for homosexuals the same rights other Canadians took for granted. For example, in 1992 a lesbian named Michelle Douglas took the Canadian Armed Forces to court for discrimination. She won her case, forcing the military to change its policy of not hiring and promoting gays and lesbians. In 1995, two elderly gay men from Vancouver Island — Jim Egan and Jack Nesbit, who had lived together for several decades — sued the federal government for the right to claim a spousal pension under the Old Age Security program. Four years later, in 1999, the Supreme Court ruled that same-sex couples were entitled to the same benefits and obligations as heterosexual common-law couples, and equal access to benefits from social programs to which they contributed.

In 1994, the Supreme Court of Canada led the world in ruling that gays and lesbians might apply for refugee status if they had been persecuted for their sexual orientation. In 1995, the Supreme Court ruled that "sexual orientation" must be "read in" to the Canadian Charter of Rights and Freedoms. In 1996, "sexual orientation" was added to the Canadian Human Rights Act, an anti-discrimination law that applies to federally regulated activities throughout Canada.

In addition to the federal Canadian Human Rights Act, each Canadian province and territory has its own human rights act to cover non-federal matters, and rights in these areas must reflect the values of the Charter of Rights and Freedoms. When the Province of Alberta excluded homosexuals from its human rights act, the Supreme Court of Canada overrode the Alberta government, ruling that protection for Alberta's homosexual citizens must be included in the act.

In 2003, Parliament passed bill C-250 to add "sexual orientation" to a section of the Criminal Code that prohibits the incitement of hatred against people based on their colour, race, religion or ethnic origin. It was obvious that a change in the law was desperately needed. When Vancouver police examined the records of crimes against groups protected by this law, they found that 62 percent of the criminal cases involving these groups were based on sexual orientation. So far, Saskatchewan is the only province whose rights arbiters have labelled as hate speech those biblical passages declaring homosexuality a sin.

Some school districts have now adopted their own anti-hate rules. The Victoria, B.C., school board adopted in 2003 a ground-breaking discrimination policy and a set of recommendations aimed at fostering respect, tolerance and safety for students with minority sexual orientations. The Vancouver, B.C., school district followed suit and in 2006 went even further by signing an agreement with two gay teachers to give them a significant voice in the revision of classroom lessons so that these would include recognition of gay, lesbian, bisexual and transgendered people. The school district also agreed to create a new social justice course — to include teachings about sexual orientation — for interested Grade 12 students.

Gay federal employees in Canada now have all the same benefits as other common-law pairs. Canadian homosexuals can bring a foreign partner to Canada permanently as long as they've been "conjugal partners" for one year. Same-sex partners have the same right to spousal support, guardianship, pensions and medical decision-making as heterosexual couples. Gay parents may adopt children. In federal prisons, Correctional Services Canada is now required to provide transsexuals with sex reassignment surgery recommended by a doctor. (The change resulted from a court ruling that a blanket ban on such surgery is discriminatory because prisons are required to provide essential health care to inmates.)

But the biggest victory of all for sexual minorities in Canada came in 2005, when Canada became the second country in the world after the Netherlands officially to sanction gay marriage nationwide. The Supreme Court ruling followed one of the hottest public debates in recent Canadian memory, led by the religious right and the conservative Canadian Alliance Party. The Pope himself announced that gay marriage must be fought with every fibre. Canadian priests urged their parishioners to contact the Prime Minister and their Members of Parliament, pressing them to oppose gay marriage because marriage was for procreation and homosexuals couldn't procreate. Pat Johnson, a columnist in the *Vancouver Courier*, commented that "if taken seriously, it [the notion of marriage only for procreation] would preclude Catholic weddings involving many paraplegics and all menopausal women, vasectomied grooms or hysterectomied brides." (It would also have precluded Catholic weddings for infertile couples and for the many people who had no intention of having children.)

Catholic Archbishop Adam Exner in Vancouver decided to sever ties with VanCity, a local credit union that had been offering educational programs to four Catholic schools. Exner's decision was based on VanCity's sponsorship of a gay and lesbian film festival — one of several of the credit union's contributions to the arts — and to its marketing campaign's inclusion of large newspaper ads featuring two men sitting together saying, "I want to bank with people who value all partnerships." Bruce Ralston, the chair of VanCity's board, reported that 85 percent of the emails and phone messages they'd received in response to the Catholic Church's initiative had been supportive of VanCity.

The anti-gay-marriage people argued that allowing gays to marry would demean the institution of marriage because gay relationships were less durable. In response, pro-gay-marriage people pointed out that in Denmark, homosexual divorces occur only 20 percent as frequently as heterosexual divorces, taking into account their population numbers. Moreover, with 37 percent of straight marriages in Canada ending in divorce and the number of common-law partnerships increasing, heterosexuals were hardly in a position to criticize the instability of gay unions.

As the debate rolled on, Canadian public opinion became more evenly divided on the issue of gay marriage, but it was clear from the polling statistics that younger Canadians were still overwhelmingly in favour. Polling had shown that those likeliest to oppose gay marriage were male, rural, over 55 years old, having high school or less education, and religious. Nonetheless, many religious people, especially Catholics, actually supported gay marriage: An Environics poll at the time found 57 percent of Canadian Catholics in favour and 40 percent opposed. Among Protestants there was only 38 percent support, with 58 percent opposed.

Globe and Mail columnist Michael Valpy weighed in to the debate with his observation that, until a few hundred years before, marriage had been a secular event and therefore the Christian church's proprietary claim to marriage and its definition in Western society was a manifestation of fudged history.

No priest is recorded officiating at a wedding in the Bible. Early Hebrew law, from which Christianity descends, presented marriage as a commercial transaction: a wife was basically purchased. The Bible is blatantly contradictory on divorce.

Nothing in the Bible prescribes monogamy or, for that matter, proscribes polygamy, which is mentioned without censure more often than the Bible alludes to homosexuality.

The Christian church's definition of marriage comes from the legal *Digesta* of the Roman emperor Justinian (483-563): Marriage is a union of a man and woman, and a communion of the whole of life.

Other writers claimed that only conservative gay people wanted the right to marry anyway; more radical gays eschewed marriage because it was a heterosexual institution. Columnist and gay man Victor Dwyer asked, tongue-in-cheek: "Who took the fun, and the fire, out of being homosexual? Wasn't it the plan of gay liberation to forge an exciting new world different from the world of straights?" Observing that straight and gay men were becoming more similar, Dwyer plaintively asked, "Should gays now dress and dance as badly as other men? Will straight guys have to listen to Liza Minnelli and Barbra Streisand?" Dwyer noted his discomfort that Canadian political leaders and other people were falling over one another to express their support for gay marriage:

And it's not just a bunch of out-of-touch political elites that are ushering us into the straight fold. When I go to family reunions in rural Ontario, my dozens of relatives extend open arms to both me and my partner of 21 years. When we moved into our Toronto neighbourhood, where working-class, hyphenated Canadians in extended families are the norm, not a single neighbour batted an eyelash. It wasn't long before they were bringing us tomatoes from their gardens and passing homemade wine over the fence. How can we stay radical and fire-breathing when you treat us like that?

Prime Minister Paul Martin declared publicly that, despite being a Catholic, he would put his duty as a legislator ahead of his religion in supporting same-sex marriage. "We are a country where there is a division of church and state," Martin told CanWest News. Churches were pleased that the new law included a provision giving them the right to refuse to conduct gay marriage ceremonies if they didn't approve of them.

LEGAL RIGHTS FOR SEXUAL MINORITIES ELSEWHERE

In 2006, an attempt to stage the first gay-pride march in Moscow ended in violence and mass arrests. Most other Western countries, however, have now moved toward legal protection for sexual minorities, though the extent of such rights still varies considerably from country to country.

In 2001, the Netherlands led the way for completely equal legal rights, including marriage and adoption. The Royal Dutch Air Force now requires everyone entering the force to undergo sensitivity training regarding homosexuals in its ranks.

The Scandinavian countries — Norway, Sweden, Denmark — have also taken a progressive stance toward homosexual rights: Norway was the first country in the world to enact a law to prevent discrimination against homosexuals (1981); Sweden the first to pass laws protecting the social service, taxes and inheritance of gays and lesbians (1988); Denmark the first to enact registered partnership laws (comparable to civil union) for same-sex couples, with most of the same rights as marriage (1989). Norway and Sweden followed suit, so that for several years civil unions for gays and lesbians have been available in all three Scandinavian countries. Gay adoption is legal only in Sweden, but Norway, Denmark and Iceland all allow "stepchild adoption," which permits a partner in a civil union to adopt the other's child.

The European Union's anti-discrimination policy has spurred reform all over continental Europe. Belgium has had gay marriage and adoption since 2003; France and Germany have both enshrined same-sex domestic partnerships in law. France still does not permit gays and lesbians to adopt, but Germany allows "stepchild adoptions." Germany now allows gays into the military and is building a memorial to the more than 10,000 homosexuals whom the Nazis deported to concentration camps, where few survived.

Italy's definition of a family has been broadened to include "a group of cohabiting persons tied by bonds of affection." Austria's Court ruled that having a higher age of sexual consent for homosexuals violated the European Convention of Human Rights.

In the UK, partly as the result of public pressure and partly because of rulings by the European Court of Human Rights, a string of improvements has occurred in recent years. Britain's M15 spy agency lifted its ban on homosexuals. Immigration policy changed to allow a foreign same-sex partner of a British citizen to obtain a residency permit. The Defence Ministry lifted its ban on gays' serving in the military and issued new guidelines allowing soldiers who have sex-change operations to remain in the army. (The Ministry also agreed to pay about four million pounds to gay and lesbian service personnel who had sued the government for wrongful dismissal.) The House of Lords ruled that anyone persecuted in another country for sexual identity could seek asylum in the UK. And in 2005, the Greater London Authority became the first public organization in the country officially to recognize same-sex couples: "civil partnership" ceremonies for both gay and straight common-law couples, granting the same rights as married couples have in everything but name, are held in the London Authority's visitors' center on Wednesdays and Saturdays; up to 25 guests may attend. The Church of England has refused to bless these unions, on the grounds that "they could erode the traditional definition of marriage." To reinforce that point, Anglican bishops voted to encourage only "sexually abstinent friendships" between people of the same sex. A British lesbian couple who had married in Canada decided to test the English law that had ruled their marriage illegal in Britain, but their appeal was defeated. Meanwhile, the Scottish court ruled that same-sex couples have the same parental rights as married heterosexual couples; a lesbian or gay couple in Scotland is now legally regarded as a "family unit." Scotland also now has a lower age of consent (14) for gay males; elsewhere in Britain it is 16 for all, except in Northern Ireland, where it is 17.

Australia has lagged behind other Western countries in enacting laws to protect the rights of sexual minorities, and in 2004, the Australian government moved to ban gay marriage, calling a union of man and woman "the commonly accepted definition of a marriage." A few years ago a federal bill amended the Broadcast Services regulations to block "offensive material" on the Internet, with heavy fines for noncompliance, providing the legal foundation for a mass of complaints against lesbian and gay websites. In 2003, the U.N. Human Rights Committee found Australia to be in breach of the International Covenant on Civil and Political Rights after it refused to grant a survivor's pension to a gay man whose partner of 38 years had died after a long military career. On a more positive note, in 2003, the Australian Legislative Assembly voted to allow same-sex couples to adopt children (although gay marriage is still banned).

There is no federal anti-discrimination law in Australia, but almost all Australian states have some such law, though what it covers varies considerably. No states or territories have anti-sodomy laws, but several states protect only "lawful sexual activity," the definition of which can vary. Some states have now granted some rights to gay and lesbian couples, but none guarantees full partnership rights. Tasmania has recognized same-sex domestic partnerships under common law, giving partners rights in making decisions about each other's health, guardianship when one partner is incapacitated, and equal access to each other's public sector pensions. The state of South Australia has now granted same-sex couples the same rights as other common-law couples in areas such as superannuation benefits and funeral and medical rights, but rights to adoption and access to reproductive technology are excluded.

New Zealand offers more protection for sexual minorities than Australia, in large part because of its national gay rights law banning discrimination in employment, education, housing, services, partnerships and other areas. The age of sexual consent is 16 for all. Lesbians and gays are allowed in the military. Lesbian couples, like straight women, have access to state-funded fertility treatments. Homosexual couples who have been together for three years enjoy the same property rights as married and common-law heterosexual couples.

Even conservative Singapore has made some tentative moves toward gay rights. The government will now hire gays for certain positions if they declare their sexual orientation when applying for work. Homosexual acts remain officially illegal, but there are now a few gay bars operating openly, and several saunas now cater almost exclusively to gay clients.

FAMILIARITY BREEDS TOLERANCE

A while ago, getting my hair cut, I noticed a man among the previously all-female staff. When I commented on this to Susan, the young woman cutting my hair, she bent toward my ear and whispered, "That's Glen. He's gay, and he is so-o-o much fun! I come from Kamloops [a small town in the B.C. Interior], and I never really knew a gay person before. I used to hear kids at my high school talking about gays, and I thought they must be awful, but Glen is really nice. And he's got an amazing sense of humour. Everybody here really likes him."

Glen probably wasn't aware that he was making a political statement when he didn't try to hide his gay identity. But in doing so, he raised the consciousness of all his co-workers, many of whom, like Susan, may never have known a gay person. As research has repeatedly shown that the strongest predictor of tolerance toward homosexuality is knowing a gay person, coming out of the closet is not only a personal step but also an important political act. In addition, it's a significant health benefit: An important American study confirmed earlier research about the positive health effects of disclosing one's gay sexual orientation to co-workers. Gay men and lesbians who felt safe to be "out" at work showed better psychological adjustment and life satisfaction, whereas those who hid their sexual orientation had high levels of anxiety and exhaustion, and feelings of shame and alienation.

Psychology professor Bob Altemeyer of the University of Manitoba wanted to test the theory that learning someone was gay would increase acceptance of gays in general, so he told his Introductory Psychology students one year that he was a homosexual and active in the gay movement. As expected, the students' opinions of him dropped a little, compared to a control group, but on the other hand, evaluations of homosexuals in general rose significantly. Altemeyer, who actually isn't gay, also presented his students with scientific findings about the biological influence on homosexuality. Afterwards, an informal survey of the students showed that nearly all of them felt that gays could not be morally faulted for their sexual orientation.

Sometimes, changes in public attitudes are most evident in small things. One recent June, the "month of brides," the Hudson's Bay Company in Vancouver had an interesting window display advertising its wedding registry service. Below the two large bride and groom mannequins, a long procession of doll-size couples of various ethnic origins, all clad in wedding finery, wound across the floor and up the back of the display. It was my four-year-old granddaughter who noticed that not all of the couples were opposite-sex: "Look, grandma," she cried excitedly, "some of the weddings are two Barbies and some are two Kens!" When questioned about the display, officials at the Bay explained matter-of-factly that it merely reflected the cultural variety that is now Vancouver, "a nod ... to those different parts of humanity that make up our customer base," and a reflection of the

Canadian demographic. The same month an editorial in the *Globe and Mail* said it another way: "On college campuses, in inner cities and across suburban neighbourhoods, men and women of all races and sexualities live, work and make love without stigma attached. The gay or mixed-race couple, who only a generation ago would have raised eyebrows if they moved in next door, go unnoticed today. Canadian society is becoming blissfully blind."

The increasing visibility of gay men and women in television and films is introducing millions of viewers in North America and elsewhere to positive examples of gays and lesbians for the first time. Coincidentally, young people are declaring their homosexuality at earlier ages. Psychologist Ritch Savin-Williams of Cornell, who has been studying gay teenagers for more than two decades, reported that in 1980 the average American gay man came out of the closet in his 20s; by 1998, the average age had dropped to 16; today the average age of first same-sex contact is 14 for boys and 16 for girls. Many of these young people are now involved in "gay-straight alliances," school clubs for gay and gay-friendly students. By 2007, over 4,000 of these clubs had formed in American and Canadian high schools.

As more and more gays and lesbians openly acknowledge their sexual orientation to their families, friends, co-workers and others, approval of sexual minorities is bound to grow. Heterosexuals will discover that gays, lesbians, bisexuals, transsexuals, cross-dressers and intersexuals are just ordinary, everyday people — the kids down the street, the couple next door, their children's teachers, the people sitting beside them in church, the lawyers handling the sales of their houses — normal people who were described in an *Economist* review as merely "sexually left-handed."

Am I too optimistic? I don't think so. The white mainstream has already discovered, at least in some countries, that people of colour are "just plain folks" — an achievement that was unimaginable in my childhood, when blacks were banished from all Vancouver hotels except one, Jews were precluded from home ownership in

West Vancouver's posh British Properties area, central Europeans were known as "bohunks," and Chinese, Japanese and East Indian Canadians were called "Chinks," "Japs" and "Ragheads." I could never have imagined then that, within my lifetime, I would live in a Canada where children of every religion, colour and ethnic background would hang out together at school and go home to parents who were legally guaranteed equal treatment and protection from discrimination and insult. I would never have predicted that one of my children would marry a Jew and another a black man, and that nobody would raise an eyebrow. Why then should I not be optimistic that we will learn to accept sexual diversity as fully as racial, ethnic and cultural diversity?

This book has reviewed some of the research on the various sexual groups that have been identified so far. But because sexology is still in its infancy, there is much, much more to discover. As research about sexual variation accumulates, we will learn that sexual diversity applies to all of us, not just to "them." We will understand that our own individual sexualities, no matter how we may label them, are all just points in a vast sexual mosaic, each one of us a unique and normal variant in the marvellous panoply of human sexual behaviour.

Acknowledgements

I N WRITING THIS BOOK, I was very fortunate to have the help and support of my family and friends. Christopher, Lise and Erica Johnson all read sections of the manuscript and gave me their frank and thoughtful criticisms as well as much loving encouragement. Beryl Young, Aida Davis, Michelle Soucie and Laura and Martin Toren critiqued various chapters and all provided helpful feedback. I am especially indebted to my friend Tamara Turner for her impressive research skills, her generous sharing of knowledge and her superb sense of humour. Most of all, I am grateful to my husband, Ross, who supported me in so many ways and was unstinting with his thoughtful comments, his cheerful confidence in both me and the book, and his many practical aids.

I very much appreciated the help I received from the librarians at UBC's Woodward Biomedical and Koerner libraries, and from those at the Vancouver Public Library.

I enjoyed working with my Raincoast editors, Derek Fairbridge and Naomi Wittes Reichstein, both of whom were sharp, organized and cheerfully supportive. I wish also to thank my agent, Carolyn Swayze, for her patience, her knowledge and her diligence.

Finally, I owe a large debt of thanks to those who so honestly and generously shared their stories with me: Danielle Anderson, "Isabella," David Harrison, Alison Brewin and Vanessa Jacobson, Byron Chiefmoon and Stanley Alexander and their children Daffney, Agatha and Davy. I feel privileged to have been allowed into your lives and your homes.

Bibliography

CHAPTER 1

Archer, Bert. *The End of Gay*. Toronto: Doubleday Canada, 1999.

Bagemihl, Bruce. *Biological Exuberance*. New York: St. Martin's Press, 1999.

Berenbaum, Sheri A. "Effects of early androgens on sex-typed activities and interests in adolescents with congenital adrenal hyperplasia." *Hormones and Behavior*, Vol. 35 (1999) 102–110.

http://www.blockbonobofoundation.org.

Brans, Jo. *Mother, I Have Something to Tell You*. New York: Doubleday, 1987.

Brown, W. M. "Masculinized finger length ratios in humans with congenital adrenal hyperplasia." *Hormones and Behavior*, Vol. 39 (2001) 325–326.

Clarke, I. J. "The sexual behavior of pre-natally androgenized ewes observed in the field." *Journal of Reproduction & Fertility*, Vol. 49 (1977) 311–315.

Collaer, Marcia L. and Melissa Hines. "Human behavioral sex differences: A role for gonadal hormones during early development." *Psychological Bulletin*, Vol. 118, No. 1 (1995) 55–107.

Diamond, Milton, Teresa Binstock and James V. Kohl. "From fertilization to adult sexual behavior." *Hormones and Behavior*, Vol. 30 (1996) 333–353.

Dittmann, Ralf W. "Sexual behavior and sexual orientation in females with congenital adrenal hyperplasia." In Lee Ellis and Linda Ebertz, eds., *Sexual Orientation*. Westport, Conn.: Praeger (1997) 53–69.

Ehrhardt, Anke A. et al. "Sexual orientation after prenatal exposure to exogenous estrogen." *Archives of Sexual Behavior*, Vol. 14, No. 1 (1985) 57–75.

Fausto-Sterling, Anne. *Myths of Gender*. New York: Basic Books, 1985.

Fitch, Roslyn Holly and Victor H. Denenberg. "A role for ovarian hormones in sexual differentiation in the brain." *Behavioural and Brain Sciences*, Vol. 23, No. 3 (1998) 311–352.

Gooren, Louis. "Biomedical theories of sexual orientation: a critical examination." In David P. McWhirter, Stephanie A. Sanders and June M. Reinisch, eds. *Homosexuality/Heterosexuality*. New York: Oxford University Press (1990) 71–77.

Gorski, Roger A. "Development of the cerebral cortex: XV. Sexual differentiation of the central nervous system." *Journal of the American Academy of Child and Adolescent Psychiatry*, Vol. 38:3 (March 1999) 344–346.

Goy, Robert W., Fred B. Bercovitch and Mary C. McBrair. "Behavioral masculinization is independent of genital masculinization in prenatally androgenized rhesus macaques." *Hormones and Behavior*, Vol. 22 (1988) 552–571.

Hines, Melissa "Hormonal and neural correlates of sex-typed behavioral development in human beings." In M. Haug et al., eds., *The Development of Sex Differences and Similarities in Behaviour (1993)*. Kluwer Academic Publishers, Netherlands, 131–149.

Hines, Melissa and Carl Shipley. "Prenatal exposure to diethylstilbestrol (DES) and the development of sexually dimorphic cognitive abilities and cerebral lateralization." *Developmental Psychology*, Vol. 20, No. 1 (1984) 81–94.

Hines, Melissa, S. F. Ahmed and I. A. Huges. "Psychological outcomes and gender-related development in complete androgen insensitivity syndrome." *Archives of Sexual Behavior*, Vol. 32, No. 2 (2003) 93–101.

Imperato-McGinley, Julianne et al. "Androgens and the evolution of male-gender identity among male pseudohermaphrodites with 5-alpha reductase deficiency." *The New England Journal of Medicine*, Vol. 300, No. 22 (May 31, 1979) 1233–1237.

Katz, Jonathan Ned. *The Invention of Heterosexuality*. London: Penguin, 1995.

McWhirter, David P., Stephanie A. Sanders and June M. Reinisch, eds. *Homosexuality/Heterosexuality*. New York: Oxford University Press (1990) 71–77.

Moir, Anne and David Jessel. *Brain Sex*. London: Penguin, 1989.

Money, John. *Gay, Straight and In-Between*. New York: Oxford University Press, 1988.

Pert, Candace B. *Molecules of Emotion*. New York: Scribner, 1997.

Roselli, Charles E., John Resko and Fred Stormshak. "Hormonal influences on sexual partner preferences in rams." *Archives of Sexual Behavior*, Vol. 31, No. 1 (2002) 43–49.

Scheirs, J. G. M. and A. J. J. M. Vingerhoets. "Handedness and other laterality indices in women prenatally exposed to DES." *Journal of Clinical and Experimental Neuropsychology*, Vol. 17, No. 5 (1995) 725–730.

Smith, Laurel L. and Melissa Hines. "Language lateralization and handedness in women prenatally exposed to diethylstilbestrol (DES)." *Psychoneuroendocrinology*, Vol. 25 (2000) 497–512.

Vasey, Paul L. "Sexual partner preference in female Japanese macaques." *Archives of Sexual Behavior*, Vol. 31, No. 1 (2002) 51–62.

Whalen, R. E. "Animal sexual differentiation: The early days and current questions." In M. Haug et al., eds. *The Development of Sex Differences and Similarities in Behavior*. Netherlands: Kluwer Academic Publishers (1993) 77–86.

CHAPTER 2

Annis, Barbara. *Same Words, Different Language*. Toronto: Penguin Canada, 2003.

Baron-Cohen, Simon. *The Essential Difference*. New York: Basic Books, 2003.

Berg, S. J. and K. E. Wynne-Edwards. "Changes in testosterone, cortisol and estradiol level in men becoming fathers." *Mayo Clinic Proceedings*, Vol. 76, No. 6 (June 2001) 582–592.

Bizendine, Louann. *The Female Brain*. New York: Morgan Road Books, 2006.

Breedlove, S. Marc. "Sex on the brain." *Nature*, Vol. 389 (23 Oct. 1997) 801.

Buss, David M. *The Dangerous Passion*. New York: Bloomsbury, 2000.

Buss, David M. *The Evolution of Desire*. New York: Basic Books, 1994.

Canli, T. et al. "Sex differences in the neural basis of emotional memories." *Proceedings of the National Academy of Sciences USA*, Vol. 99, No. 16 (2002) 10789–10794.

Collaer, Marcia L. and Melissa Hines. "Human behavioral sex differences: A role for gonadal hormones during early development?" *Psychological Bulletin*, Vol. 118, No. 1 (1995) 55–107.

Collins, D. W. and D. Kimura. "A large sex difference on a two-dimensional mental rotation task." *Behavioral Neuroscience*, Vol. 111 (1997) 845–849.

Connellan, H. et al. "Sex differences in human neonatal social perception." *Infant Behavior and Development*, Vol. 23 (2000) 113–118.

Emlen, Stephen T. and Peter M. Buston. "Cognitive processes underlying human mate choice: the relationship between self-perception and mate preference in western society." *Proceedings of the National Academy of Sciences*, Vol. 100, No. 15 (2003) 8805–8810.

Geary, D. et al. "Sex differences in spatial cognition, computational fluency and arithmetical reasoning." *Journal of Experimental Child Psychology*, Vol. 77 (2000) 337–353.

Giedd, Jay N. et al. "Brain development during childhood and adolescence: a longitudinal

MRI study." *Nature Neuroscience*, Vol. 2, No. 10 (Oct. 1999) 861–863.

Gorski, Roger A. "Development of the cerebral cortex: XV. Sexual differentiation of the central nervous system." *Journal of the American Academy of Child and Adolescent Psychiatry*, Vol. 38:3 (March 1999) 344–346.

Gray, John. *Men Are from Mars, Women Are from Venus*. New York: Harper Perennial, 1992.

Grimshaw, Gina M., Gabriel Sitarenios and Jo-Anne K. Finegan. "Mental rotation at seven years — relations with prenatal testosterone levels and spatial play experiences." *Brain and Cognition*, Vol. 29 (1995) 85–100.

Grimshaw, Gina M., Philip Bryden and Jo-Anne K. Finegan. "Relations between testosterone and cerebral lateralization in children." *Neuropsychology*, Vol. 9, No. 1 (1995) 68–79.

Gron, George. "Brain activation during human navigation: gender-different neural networks as substrate of performance." *Nature Neuroscience*, Vol. 3, No. 4 (April 2000) 404–408.

Gur, Ruben C. et al. "Sex differences in regional cerebral glucose metabolism during a resting state." *Science*, New Series, Vol. 267, Issue 5197 (Jan. 27 1995) 528–531.

Hampson, Elisabeth. "Variations in sex-related cognitive abilities across the menstrual cycle." *Brain and Cognition*, Vol. 14 (1990) 26–43.

Hellige, Joseph B. *Hemispheric Asymmetry: What's Right and What's Left*. Cambridge and London: Harvard University Press, 1993.

Kimura, Doreen. *Sex and Cognition*. Cambridge, Mass.: MIT Press, 1999.

Kimura, Doreen. "Body asymmetry and intellectual pattern." *Personality and Individual Differences*, Vol. 19, No. 1 (1994) 53–60.

Kimura, Doreen and Paul G. Clarke. "Cognitive pattern and dermatoglyphic asymmetry." *Personality and Individual Differences* (Dec. 30, 2001) 579–586.

Lacreuse, Agnes et al. "Spatial cognition in rhesus monkeys: male superiority declines with age." *Hormones and Behavior*, Vol. 36 (1999) 70–76.

Legato, Marianne. *Eve's Rib: The New Science of Gender-Specific Medicine and How It Can Save Your Life*. New York: Harmony Books, 2002.

Lippa, Richard A. "Handedness, sexual orientation and gender-related personality traits in men and women." *Archives of Sexual Behavior*, Vol. 32, No. 2 (2003) 103–114.

Lutchmaya, S. and S. Baron-Cohen. "Human sex differences in social and non-social looking preferences at 12 months of age." *Infant Behaviour and Development*, Vol. 25, No. 3 (2002) 319–325.

Lutchmaya, S., S. Baron-Cohen and P. Raggatt. "Foetal testosterone and vocabulary size in 18- and 24-month-old infants." *Infant Behaviour and Development*, Vol. 24, No. 4 (2002) 418–424.

Marano, Hara E. "The New Sex Scorecard." *Psychology Today*, July/August 2003.

Meltzoff, Andrew N. and Patricia Kuhl. *The Scientist in the Crib.* New York: William Morrow & Co., 1999.

Nelson, Charles A. and Floyd E. Bloom. "Child development and neuroscience." *Child Development*, Vol. 68, No. 5 (1997) 970–987.

Phillips, Micheal D. "Temporal lobe activation demonstrates sex-based differences during passive listening." *Radiology*, Vol. 220 (2001) 202–207.

Sanders, Geoff and Anjela Kadam, "Prepubescent children show the adult relationship between dermatoglyphic asymmetry and performance on sexually dimorphic tasks." *Cortex*, Vol. 37 (2001) 91–100.

Sanders, Geoff, F. Aubert and A. Kadam. "Asymmetries in finger ridge count correlate with performance on sexually dimorphic tasks in children and adults." *International Academy of Sex Research*, XXI Annual Meeting (1995) 20–24.

Schmitt, David. "Universal sex differences in the desire for sexual variety." *Journal of Personality and Social Psychology*, Vol. 85, No. 1 (2003) 85–104.

Shaywitz, Sally and Bennett. "Sex differences in the functional organization of the brain for language." *Nature*, Vol. 373 (1995) 607–9.

Skaletsky, Helen et al. "The male-specific region of the human Y chromosome is a mosaic of discrete sequence classes." *Nature*, Vol. 423 (June 19, 2003) 825.

Sullivan, Andrew. "The He hormone." *The New York Times Magazine* (April 9, 2000) 46–79.

Swaab, D. F. L. G. Gooren and M. A. Hofman. "Brain research, gender, and sexual orientation." *Journal of Homosexuality*, Vol. 28, 3–4 (1995) 283–301.

Tannen, Deborah. *You Just Don't Understand: Women and Men in Conversation.* New York: Ballantine Books, 1990.

Van Goozen, Stephanie H. M. et al. "Gender differences in behaviour: activating effects of cross-sex hormones." *Psychoneuroendocrinology*, Vol. 20, No. 4 (1995) 343–363.

Wedekind, Claus et al. "MHC-dependent mate preferences in humans." *Proceedings of the Royal Society of London*, Vol. 260 (1995) 245–249.

Whalley, Laurence J. *The Aging Brain.* New York: Columbia University Press, 2001.

Witelson, S. F., D. L. Kigar and H. J. Stoner-Beresh. "Sex differences in the numerical density of neurons in the pyramidal layers of human prefrontal cortex: a stereologic study." *Society for Neuroscience Abstracts*, Vol. 27 (Programme No. 80.18) 2001.

Yang, Jerry et al. "Aberrant patterns of X chromosome inactivation in bovine clones." *Nature Genetics*, Vol. 31 (2002) 216–220.

CHAPTER 3

Bailey, J. M. et al. "Butch, femme, or straight acting? Partner preferences of gay men and lesbians." *Journal of Personality & Social Psychology*, Vol. 73, No. 5 (1997) 960–973.

Baumeister, Roy F. "Gender differences in erotic plasticity: The female sex drive as socially flexible and responsive." *Psychological Bulletin*, Vol. 126, No. 3 (2000) 347–374.

Bell, Alan P. and Martin S. Weinberg. *Homosexualities*. New York: Simon and Shuster, 1978.

Blanchard, Ray, I. G. Racansky and Betty W. Steiner. "Phallometric detection of fetishistic arousal in heterosexual male cross-dressers." *The Journal of Sex Research*, Vol. 22, No. 4 (1986) 452–462.

Blumstein, Philip and Pepper Schwartz. *American Couples*. New York: William Morrow, 1983.

Bogaert, Anthony F. "Physical development and sexual orientation in women: Height, weight and age of puberty comparisons." *Personality and Individual Differences*, Vol. 24, No. 1 (1998) 115–121.

Bogaert, Anthony F. and Ray Blanchard. "Physical development and sexual orientation in men: Height, weight and age of puberty differences." *Personality and Individual Differences*, Vol. 21, No. 1 (1996) 77–84.

Burana, Lila and Roxxie and Linnea Due. *Dagger on Butch Women*. Pittsburgh: Cleis Press, 1994.

Charbonneau, C. and P. S. Lander. "Redefining sexuality: Women becoming lesbian in midlife." In B. Sang, ed. *Lesbians at Midlife: The Creative Transition*. San Francisco: Spinsters Books (1991) 35–43.

Diamond, Lisa M. and Ritch Savin-Williams. "Explaining diversity in the development of same-sex sexuality among young women." *Journal of Social Issues*, Vol. 56, No. 2 (2000) 297–313.

Diamond, Milton. "Homosexuality and bisexuality in different populations." *Archives of Sexual Behavior*, Vol. 22, No. 4 (1993) 291–311.

Faderman, Lillian. *Surpassing the Love of Men*. New York: William Morrow, 1981.

Fassinger, Ruth E. and Susan L. Morrow. "Overcome: Repositioning lesbian sexualities." In Louis Diamont and Richard D. McAnulty, eds., *The Psychology of Sexual Orientation, Behavior and Identity*. Westport, Conn.: Greenwood Press (1995) 197–219.

Flaks, David K. et al. "Lesbians choosing motherhood: A comparative study of lesbian and heterosexual parents and their children." *Developmental Psychology*, Vol. 31, No. 1 (1995) 103–114.

Gagnon, John H., Cathy Stein Greenblat and Michael Kimmel. "Bisexuality: A sociological perspective." In Erwin H. Haeberle and Rolf Gindorf, eds., *Bisexualities*. New York: Continuum (1998) 81–105.

Golombok, Susan et al. "Children with lesbian parents: a community study." *Developmental Psychology*, Vol. 39, No. 1 (2003) 20–33.

Gould, Terry. *The Lifestyles*. Toronto: Random House of Canada, 1999.

Green, Richard. "Sexual identity of 37 children raised by homosexual or transsexual parents." *American Journal of Psychiatry*, Vol. 135, No. 6 (1978) 692–697.

Herdt, Gilbert. "Bisexuality and the causes of homosexuality: the case of the Sambia." In Erwin H. Haeberle and Rolf Gindorf, eds., Bisexualities. New York: Continuum (1998).

Herdt, Gilbert. Third Sex, Third Gender. New York: Zone Books, 1994.

Isay, Richard A. "Psychoanalytic theory and the therapy of gay men." In David P. McWhirter, Stephanie Sanders and June M. Reinisch, eds. Homosexuality/Heterosexuality. New York: Oxford University Press (1990) 283–303.

Katz, Jonathan Ned. Gay American History. New York: Crowell, 1976.

Kaye, Marcia. "Women with Women." Homemakers, June 2003, 46–51.

Kinsey, Alfred. Sexual Behavior in the Human Female. Philadelphia: W. B. Saunders, 1953.

Kinsey, Alfred. Sexual Behavior in the Human Male. Philadelphia: W. B. Saunders, 1948.

Kitzinger, Celia. "Transitions from heterosexuality to lesbianism: the discursive production of lesbian identities." Developmental Psychology, Vol. 31, No. 1 (1995) 95–104.

Laumann, Edward O. et al. The Social Organization of Sexuality: Sexual Practices in the United States. University of Chicago Press, 1994.

Lippa, Richard A. "Gender-related traits of heterosexual and homosexual men and women." Archives of Sexual Behavior, Vol. 31, No. 1 (2002) 83–98.

Loulan, JoAnn. Lesbian Passion. San Francisco: Spinsters/Aunt Lute, 1987.

Loulan, JoAnn. Lesbian Sex. San Francisco: Spinsters Ink, 1984.

McKnight, Jim. Straight Science? London and New York: Routledge, 1997.

Money, John. Gay, Straight and In-Between. New York: Oxford University Press, 1988.

Patterson, Charlotte J. "Lesbian mothers, gay fathers and their children." In Anthony R. D'Augelli, ed., Lesbian, Gay and Bisexual Identities over the Lifespan. New York: Oxford University Press (1995) 262–290.

Pillard, Richard. "The Kinsey scale: is it familial?" In David P. McWhirter, Stephanie Sanders and June M. Reinisch, eds. Homosexuality/Heterosexuality. New York: Oxford University Press (1990) 88–100.

Rosenbluth, S. "Is sexual orientation a matter of choice?" Psychology of Women Quarterly, Vol. 21 (1997) 595–610.

Siegelman, Marvin. "Parental backgrounds of homosexual and heterosexual men: a cross national replication." Archives of Sexual Behavior, Vol. 10, No. 6 (1981) 505–513.

Strickland, Bonnie R. "Research on sexual orientation and human development: a commentary." Developmental Psychology, Vol. 31, No. 1 (1995) 137–140.

Symons, D. The Evolution of Human Sexuality. New York: Oxford University Press, 1979.

VanWyk, Paul H. and Chrisann S. Geist. "Psychosocial development of heterosexual, bisexual and homosexual behavior." Archives of Sexual Behavior, Vol. 13, No. 6 (1984) 505–544.

Vidal, Gore. Palimpsest. New York: Random House, 1995.

Weinrich, James D. *Sexual Landscapes*. New York: Scribner's, 1987.

Whitham, Frederick L. and Robin M. Mathy. *Male Homosexuality in Four Societies*. New York: Praeger, 1985.

Whitham, Frederick et al. "The emergence of lesbian sexuality and identity cross-culturally: Brazil, Peru, the Philippines, and the United States." *Archives of Sexual Behavior*, Vol. 27, No. 1 (1998) 31–56.

Swaab, D. F. and M. A. Hofman. "Sexual differentiation of the human hypothalamus in relation to gender and sexual orientation." *Trends in Neurosciences*, Vol. 18 (1995) 64–270.

CHAPTER 4

Beemer, Blaine R. "Gender dysphoria update." *Journal of Psychosocial Nursing*, Vol. 34, No. 4 (1996) 12–19.

Calipinto, John. *As Nature Made Him*. Toronto: Harper Collins, 2000.

Chivers, Meredith L. and J. Michael Bailey. "Sexual orientation of female-to-male transsexuals: A comparison of homosexual and nonhomosexual types." *Archives of Sexual Behavior*, Vol. 29, No. 3 (2000) 259–278.

Coleman, Eli. "Paradigmatic changes in the understanding of bisexuality." In Erwin H. Haeberle and Rolf Gindorf, eds. *Bisexualities*. New York: Continuum (1998) 107–117.

Devor, Holly. FTM: *Female-to-Male Transsexuals in Society*. Bloomington, Ill.: Indiana University Press, 1997.

Diamond, Lisa M. "What does sexual orientation orient? A biobehavioral model distinguishing romantic love and sexual desire." *Psychological Review*, Vol. 110, No. 1 (2003) 73–192.

Diamond, Milton. "Bisexuality: A biological perspective." In Erwin H. Haeberle and Rolf Gindorf, eds. *Bisexualities*. Westport, Conn.: Praeger (1998) 53–79.

Diamond, Milton and Keith Sigmundson. "Sex reassignment at birth." *Archives of Pediatric and Adolescent Medicine*, Vol. 151, No. 3 (1997) 298–304.

Diamond, Milton. "Self-testing among transsexuals: A check on sexual identity." *Journal of Psychology & Human Sexuality*, Vol. 8, No. 3 (1996) 61–82.

Diamond, Milton. "Homosexuality and bisexuality in different populations." *Archives of Sexual Behavior*, Vol. 22, No. 4 (1993) 291–311.

Dicks, Grace H. and A. T. Childers. "The social transformation of a boy who lived his first fourteen years as a girl: a case history." *American Journal of Orthopsychiatry*, Vol.4, No. 4 (1934).

Dixon, Joan K. "The commencement of bisexual activity in swinging married women over age thirty." *The Journal of Sex Research*, Vol. 20, No. 1 (1984) 71–90.

Fisher, Helen E. et al. "Defining the Brain Systems of Lust, Romantic Attraction, and

Attachment." *Archives of Sexual Behavior*, Vol. 31, No. 5 (2002) 413–419.

Fox, Ronald C. "Bisexual identities." In A. R. D'Augelli and C. J. Patterson, eds., *Lesbian, Gay and Bisexual Identities Over the Lifespan: Psychological Perspectives*. New York: Oxford University Press (1995) 48–86.

Gagnon, John H., Cathy Stein Greenblat and Michael Kimmel. "Bisexuality: A sociological perspective." In Erwin J. Haeberle and Rolf Gindorf, eds. *Bisexualities*. New York: Continuum (1998) 81–105.

Garber, Marjorie. *Vice-Versa*. New York: Simon & Schuster, 1995.

Glausiusz, Josie. "Transsexual brains," *Discover*, January 1996.

Gooren, Louis. "The endocrinology of transsexualism: a review and commentary." *Psychoneuroendocrinology*, Vol. 15, No. 1 (1990) 3–14.

Gould, Terry. *The Lifestyle*. Random House Canada, 1999.

Haeberle, Erwin J. "Bisexuality: History and dimensions of a modern scientific problem." In Erwin J. Haeberle and Rolf Gindorf, eds. *Bisexualities*. New York: Continuum (1998) 13–51.

Hill, Ivan, Ed. *The Bisexual Spouse*. McLean, VA: Barlina Books, Inc., 1987.

Holmberg, Carl B. "Sexualities and popular culture." *Foundations of Popular Culture*, Vol. 6. London: Sage Publications, 1998.

Kessler, Suzanne J. *Lessons from the Intersexed*. Piscataway, NJ: Rutgers University Press, 1998.

Kuiper, Bram and Peggy Cohen-Kettenis. "Sex reassignment surgery: a study of 141 Dutch Transsexuals." *Archives of Sexual Behavior*, Vol. 17, No. 5 (1988) 439–457.

Lippa, Richard A. "Gender-related traits in transsexuals and nontranssexuals." *Archives of Sexual Behavior*, Vol. 30, No. 6 (2001) 603–614.

Peplau, Letitia Anne and Linda D. Garnets. "A new paradigm for understanding women's sexuality and sexual orientation." *Journal of Social Issues*, Vol. 56, No. 2 (2000) 329–350.

Phornphutkul, Chanika, Anne Fausto-Sterling and Philip A. Gruppuso. "Experience and reason." *Pediatrics*, Vol. 106, No. 1 (2000) 135–137.

Richards, Gwendolyn. "The double life of Frances Smith," *Globe & Mail*, July 5, 2003.

Rust, Paula C. "'Coming out' in the age of social constructionism: sexual identity formation among lesbian and bisexual women." *Gender and Society*, Vol. 7, No. 1 (Mar. 1993) 50–77.

Sadeghi, Majid and Ali Fakhrai. "Transsexualism in female monozygotic twins: a case report." *Australian and New Zealand Journal of Psychiatry*, Vol. 34, No. 5 (2000) 862–864.

Slijper, Froukje M. E. et al. "Long-term psychological evaluation of intersex children." *Archives of Sexual Behavior*, Vol. 27, No. 2 (1998) 125–144.

Snaith, Philip. "Sex reassignment surgery: A study of 141 Dutch transsexuals." *British Journal of Psychiatry*, Vol. 162 (1993) 681–685.

Vasey, Paul L. "Sexual partner preference in female Japanese macaques." *Archives of Sexual Behavior*, Vol. 31, No. 1 (2002) 51–62.

Webster, Lynne. "Female-to-male gender reassignment." *British Journal of Sexual Medicine*, Vol. 25 (May–June 1998) 8–10.

Weinberg, Martin S., Colin Williams and Douglas W. Pryor. *Dual Attraction: Understanding Bisexuality*. New York: Oxford University Press, 1994.

Weinrich, James D. *Sexual Landscapes*. New York: Scribner's, 1987.

Wolfradt, Uwe and Kerstin Neumann. "Depersonalization, self-esteem and body image in male-to-female transsexuals compared to male and female controls." *Archives of Sexual Behavior*, Vol. 30, No. 3 (2001) 301–310.

Zucker, Kenneth J. "Gender identity disorders: a developmental perspective." In Louis Diamont and Richard D. McAnulty, eds. *The Psychology of Sexual Orientation, Behaviour and Identity*. Westport, Conn.: Greenwood Press, 1995.

Zucker, Kenneth J. and Susan J. Bradley. *Gender Identity Disorder and Psychosexual Problems in Children and Adolescents*. New York/London: The Guilford Press, 1995.

CHAPTER 5

Alexander, Joel E. and Kenneth J. Sufka. "Cerebral lateralization in homosexual males: A preliminary EEG investigation." *International Journal of Psychophysiology*, Vol. 15 (1993) 269–274.

Allen, Laura S. and Roger A. Gorski. "Sexual orientation and the size of the anterior commissure in the human brain." *Proceedings of the National Academy of Science USA*, Vol. 89 (Aug. 1992) 7199–7202.

Bennett, Ruth. "Sexual orientation linked to handedness," *Science News*, July 22, 2000.

Bogaert, Anthony F. and Scott Hershberger. "The relation between sexual orientation and penile size." *Archives of Sexual Behavior*, Vol. 28, No. 3 (1999) 213–221.

Breedlove, Marc, Terrance J. Williams et al. "Finger-length ratios and sexual orientation. *Nature* Brief Communication, Vol. 404 (March 30, 2000) 455–456.

Brown, Vindy M. et al. "Differences in finger-length ratios between self-identified 'butch' and 'femme' lesbians." *Archives of Sexual Behavior*, Vol. 31, No. 1 (2002) 123–127.

Byne, William et al. "The interstitial nuclei of the human anterior hypothalamus: An investigation of variation with sex, sexual orientation, and HIV status." *Hormones and Behaviour,* Vol. 40 (2001) 86–92.

Green, Richard and Robert Young. "Hand preference, sexual preference, and transsexualism." *Archives of Sexual Behavior*, Vol. 30, No. 6 (2001) 565–574.

Hall, J. A. Y. and Doreen Kimura. "Sexual orientation and performance on sexually dimorphic motor tasks." *Archives of Sexual Behavior*, Vol. 24, No. 4 (1995) 395–407.

Hall, J. A. Y. and D. Kimura. "Dermatoglyphic asymmetry and sexual orientation in men." *Behavioral Neuroscience*, Vol. 108, No. 6 (1994) 1203–1206.

Hall, J. A. Y. and D. Kimura. "Homosexuality and circadian rhythms." *Neuropsychopharmacology*, Vol. 9 Notes (1993) 126s.

Hall, J. A. Y. and D. Kimura. "Homosexuality, cognitive abilities and the organizational hypothesis." *Society for Neuroscience Abstracts*, Vol. 18 (1992) 1210.

Hall, Lynn S. and Craig T. Love. "Finger-length ratios in female monozygotic twins discordant for sexual orientation." *Archives of Sexual Behavior*, Vol. 32, No. 1 (2003) 23–28.

Halpern, Diane F. and Marciana Crothers. "Sex, sexual orientation, and cognition." In Lee Ellis and Linda Ebertz, eds. *Sexual Orientation*. Westport, Conn.: Praeger (1997) 181–197.

Hamer, Dean. *The Science of Desire*. New York: Simon and Shuster, 1994.

Hines, M. "Hormonal and neural correlates of sex-typed behavioural development in human beings." In M. Haug et al, eds. *The Development of Sex Differences and Similarities in Behaviour*. Netherlands: Kluwer Academic Publishers (1993) 131–149.

Hu, Stella et al. "Linkage between sexual orientation and chromosome Xq28 in males but not in females." *Nature Genetics*, Vol. 11 (Nov. 1995) 248–256.

Lalumiere, Martin L., Ray Blanchard and Kenneth J. Zucker. "Sexual orientation and handedness in men and women: a meta-analysis." *Psychological Bulletin*, Vol. 126, No. 4 (2000) 575–592.

LeVay, Simon. "A difference in hypothalamic structure between heterosexual and homosexual men." *Science* (Aug. 3, 1991) 1034–1037.

LeVay, Simon. *The Sexual Brain*. Cambridge, Mass.: MIT Press (Bradford) 1993.

LeVay, Simon and Dean H. Hamer. "Evidence for biological influence in male homosexuality." In *The Scientific American Book of the Brain*, 1999.

Lindesay, James. "Laterality shift in homosexual men." *Neuropsychologia*, Vol. 25, No. 6 (1987) 965–969.

McCormick, Cheryl M. and Sandra Witelson. "Functional cerebral asymmetry in homosexual men and women." *Neuroendocrinology* Letter, Vol. 12 (1990) 300.

McCormick, Cheryl M., Sandra Witelson and Edward Kingstone. "Left-handedness in homosexual men and women: neuroendocrine implications." *Psychoneuroendocrinology*, Vol. 15, No. 1 (1990) 69–76.

McFadden, Dennis. "Masculinization effects in the auditory system." *Archives of Sexual Behavior*, Vol. 31, No. 1 (2002) 99–111.

McFadden, Dennis and Craig A. Champlin. "Comparison of auditory evoked potentials in heterosexual, homosexual, and bisexual males and females." *Journal of the Association for Research in Otolaryngology*, Vol. 1 (2000) 89–99.

McFadden, Dennis and Edward G. Pasanan. "Comparison of the auditory systems of heterosexuals and homosexuals: click-evoked otoacoustic emissions." *Proceedings of the National Academy of Science, USA*, Vol. 95 (March 1998) 2709–2713.

Mustanski, Brian, J. Michael Bailey and Sarah Kaspar. "Dermatoglyphics, handedness, sex, and sexual orientation." *Archives of Sexual Behavior*, Vol. 31, No. 1 (2002) 113–122.

Rahman, Qazi, Veena Kumari and Glenn Wilson. "Sexual orientation-related differences in prepulse inhibition of the human startle response." *Behavioral Neuroscience*, Vol. 117, No. 5 (2003) 1096–1102.

Savic, Ivanka and Hans Berglund. "Brain response to putative pheromones in homosexual men and lesbian women." *Proc. National Academy of Sciences USA*, Vol. 102, No. 20 (May 17, 2005) 7356-7361.

Swaab, D. F. and M. A. Hofman. "An enlarged suprachiasmatic nucleus in homosexual men." *Brain Research*, Vol. 537 (1990) 141–148.

Swaab, D. F. and M. A. Hofman. "Sexual differentiation of the human hypothalamus in relation to gender and sexual orientation." *Trends in Neurosciences*, Vol. 18 (1995) 264–270.

Wegesin, Domonick J. "A neuropsychologic profile of homosexual and heterosexual men and women." *Archives of Sexual Behavior*, Vol. 27, No. 1 (1998) 91–108.

Witelson, Sandra F. "Hand and sex difference in the isthmus and genu of the human corpus callosum." *Brain*, Vol. 112 (1989) 799–835.

Zucker, Kenneth J., Martin L. Lalumiere and Ray Blanchard. "Sexual orientation and handedness in men and women: a meta-analysis." *Psychological Bulletin*, Vol. 126, No. 4 (2000) 575–592.

CHAPTER 6

Bailey, J. Michael, Michael P. Dunne and Nicholas G. Martin. "Genetic and environmental influences on sexual orientation and its correlates in an Australian twin sample." *Journal of Personality and Social Psychology*, Vol. 78, No. 3 (2000) 524–536.

Bailey, J. Michael et al. "A family history study of male sexual orientation using three independent samples." *Behavior Genetics*, Vol. 29, No. 2 (Mar. 1999) 79–86.

Bailey, J. Michael "Biological perspectives on sexual orientation." In Anthony R. d'Augelli and Charlotte Patterson, eds. *Lesbian, Gay and Bisexual Identities Over the Lifespan: Psychological Perspectives*. New York: Oxford University Press (1995) 102–135.

Bailey, J. Michael and Richard C. Pillard. "Genetics of human sexual orientation," *Annual Review of Sex Research*, Vol. 6 (1995) 126–150.

Bianchi, Diana W. et al. "Male fetal progenitor cells persist in maternal blood for as long as 27 years postpartum." *Proceedings of the National Academy of Science USA*, Vol. 93 (1996) 705–707.

Blanchard, Ray et al. "Interaction of fraternal birth order and handedness in the development of male homosexuality." *Hormones and Behavior*, Vol. 49 (2006) 405-414.

Blanchard, Ray. "Quantitative and theoretical analyses of the relation between older brothers and homosexuality in men." *Journal of Theoretical Biology*, 230 (2004) 173-187.

Blanchard, Ray et al. "Fraternal birth order and birth weight in probably prehomosexual feminine boys." *Hormones and Behavior*, Vol. 41 (2002) 321-327.

Blanchard, Ray and L. Ellis. "Birth weight, sexual orientation, and the sex of preceding siblings." *Journal of Biosocial Science*, Vol. 33 (2001) 451-467.

Blanchard, Ray. "Fraternal birth order and the maternal immune hypothesis of male homosexuality." *Hormones and Behavior*, Vol. 40 (2001) 105-114.

Blanchard, Ray et al. "The relation of birth order to sexual orientation in men and women." *Journal of Biosocial Science*, Vol. 30 (1998) 511-519.

Blanchard, Ray. "Birth order and sibling sex ratio in homosexual versus heterosexual males and females." *Annual Review of Sex Research*, Vol. 8 (1997) 27-67.

Blanchard, Ray and Philip Klassen. "H-Y antigen and homosexuality in men." *Journal of Theoretical Biology*, Vol. 185 (1997) 373-378.

Blanchard, Ray et al. "Birth order and sibling sex ratio in two samples of Dutch gender-dysphoric homosexual males." *Archives of Sexual Behavior*, Vol. 25, No. 5 (1996) 495-514.

Bogaert, Anthony F. "Biological versus nonbiological older brothers and men's sexual orientation." *The National Academy of Sciences of the USA*, Vol. 103, No. 28 (July 11, 2006) 10771-10774.

Bogaert, Anthony. "Birth order and sexual orientation in a national probability sample." *The Journal of Sex Research*, Vol. 37, No. 4 (Nov.2000) 361-368.

Bogaert, Anthony. "Birth order and sibling sex ratio in homosexual and heterosexual non-white men." *Archives of Sexual Behavior*, Vol. 27, No. 5 (1998) 467.

Bogle, A. C., T. Reed and R. J. Rose. "Replication of asymmetry of a-b ridge count and behavioral discordance in monozygotic twins." *Behavior Genetics*, Vol. 24, No. 1 (1994) 65-72.

Burr, Chandler. A *Separate Creation*. New York: Hyperion, 1996.

Cantor, James M. et al. "How many gay men owe their sexual orientation to fraternal birth order?" *Archives of Sexual Behavior*, Vol. 31, No. 1 (2002) 63-71.

Dawood, Khytam et al. "Familial aspects of male homosexuality." *Archives of Sexual Behavior*, Vol. 29, No. 2 (2000) 155-163.

Frye, C. A. and L. E. Bayon. "Mating stimuli influence endogenous variations in the neurosteroids 3alpha, 5alpha-THP and 3alpha-Diol." *Journal of Neuroendocrinology*, Vol. 11, No. 11 (Nov 1999) 839-847.

Gilger, Jeffrey W. "Contributions and promise of human behavioral genetics."

Human Biology, Vol. 72, No. 1 (2000) 229–255.

Giordano, G. and M. Giusti. "Hormones and psychosexual differentiation." *Minerva Endocrinology*, Vol. 20, No. 3 (Sept 1995) 165–193.

Gooren, Louis. "Biomedical theories of sexual orientation: a critical examination." In David P. McWhirter, Stephanie A. Sanders and June M. Reinisch, eds. *Homosexuality/Heterosexuality*. New York: Oxford University Press (1990) 71–77.

Hamer, Dean and Peter Copeland. *Living With Our Genes*. New York: Doubleday, 1998.

Hamer, Dean and Peter Copeland. *The Science of Desire: The Search for the Gay Gene and the Biology of Behavior*. New York: Simon & Shuster, 1994.

Hershberger, Scott L. "A twin registry study of male and female sexual orientation." *The Journal of Sex Research*, Vol. 34, No. 2 (1997) 212–222.

Kendler, Kenneth S. et al. "Sexual orientation in a US national sample of twin and non-twin sibling pairs." *American Journal of Psychiatry*, Vol. 157 (2000) 1843–1846.

Kieler, Helle et al. "Sinistrality — a side effect of prenatal sonography: A comparative study of young men." *Epidemiology*, Vol. 12, No. 6 (2001) 618–623.

Lalumiere, Martin L., Ray Blanchard and Kenneth J. Zucker. "Sexual orientation and handedness in men and women: a meta-analysis." *Psychological Bulletin*, Vol. 126, No. 4 (2000) 575–592.

Lalumiere, Martin L., Grant T. Harris and Marnie E. Rice. "Birth order and fluctuating asymmetry: a first look." *Proceedings of the Royal Society of London*, Vol. 266 (1999) 2351–2354.

Machin, Geoffrey A. "Some causes of genotypic and phenotypic discordance in monozygotic twin pairs." *American Journal of Medical Genetics*, Vol. 61 (1996) 216–228.

McFadden, Dennis. "Masculinization effects in the auditory system." *Archives of Sexual Behavior*, Vol. 31, No. 1 (2002) 99–111.

McGue, Matt and Thomas J. Bouchard, Jr. "Genetic and environmental influences on human behavioral differences." *Annual Review of Neuroscience*, Vol. 21 (1998) 1–24.

McKnight, Jim. *Straight Science?* London and New York: Routledge, 1997.

Martin, Nicholas, Dorret Boomsma and Geoffrey Machin. "A twin-pronged attack on complex traits." *Nature Genetics*, Vol. 17 (1997) 387–392.

Miller, Edward M. "Homosexuality, birth order, and evolution: Towards an equilibrium reproductive economics of homosexuality." *Archives of Sexual Behavior*, Vol. 29, No. 1 (2000) 1–34.

Mustanski, Brian, J. Michael Bailey and Sarah Kaspar. "Dermatoglyphics, handedness, sex, and sexual orientation." *Archives of Sexual Behavior*, Vol. 31, No. 1 (2002) 113–122.

Pattatucci, Angela M. "Molecular investigations into complex behavior: lessons from sexual orientation studies." *Human Biology*, Vol. 70, No. 2 (1998) 367–386.

Pillard, Richard C. "The search for a genetic influence on sexual orientation." In Vernon A. Rosario, ed., *Science and Homosexualities*. New York: Routledge (1997) 226–241.

Purcell, David W., Ray Blanchard and Kenneth J. Zucker. "Birth order in a contemporary sample of gay men." *Archives of Sexual Behavior*, Vol. 29, No. 4 (2000) 349–356.

Puts, David A., Cynthia L. Jordan and S. Marc Breedlove. "Oh brother, where art thou? The fraternal birth-order effect on male sexual orientation." *The National Academy of Sciences of the USA*, Vol. 103, No. 28 (July 11, 2006) 10531-10532.

Schlinger, B. A., K. K. Soma and S. E. London. "Neurosteroids and brain sexual differentiation." *Trends in Neuroscience*, Vol. 24, No. 8 (2001) 429–431.

Segal, Nancy. *Entwined Lives*. London: Penguin, 1999.

Thornhill, Randy and Anders Pape Moller. "Developmental stability, disease and medicine." *Biological Reviews of the Cambridge Philosophical Society*, Vol. 72, Cambridge University Press (1997) 497–548.

Turner, William J. "Comments on discordant monozygotic twinning in homosexuality." *Archives of Sexual Behavior*, Vol. 23, No. 1 (1994) 115–119.

Weinrich, James D. "Biological research on sexual orientation: a critique of the critics." *Journal of Homosexuality*, Vol. 28 (1995) 197–213.

Yeo, Ronald A. "Developmental instability and phenotypic variation in neural organization." In N. Raz, ed., *The Other Side of the Error Term*. Amsterdam: Elsevier Science B.V., 1998.

Zucker, Kenneth J. et al. "Sibling sex ratio of boys with gender identity disorder." *Journal of Child Psychology and Psychiatry*, Vol. 38, No. 5 (1997) 543–551.

CHAPTER 7

Bem, Daryl J. "Exotic becomes erotic: A developmental theory of sexual orientation." *Psychological Review*, Vol. 103, No. 2 (1996) 320–335.

Blumstein, Philip and Pepper Schwartz. "Intimate relationships and the creation of sexuality." In David P. McWhirter, Stephanie Sanders and June M. Reinisch, eds. *Homosexuality/Heterosexuality*. New York: Oxford University Press (1990) 300–320.

Breedlove, S. Marc, Bradley M. Cooke and Cynthia L. Jordan. "The orthodox view of brain sexual differentiation." *Brain, Behavior and Evolution*, Vol. 54 (1999) 8–14.

Butler, Paul, Richard H. Mills and George J. Bloch. "Inhibition of lordosis behavior in male and female rats by androgens and progesterone." *Hormones and Behavior*, Vol. 40 (2002) 384–395.

Byne, William. "Why we cannot conclude that sexual orientation is primarily a biological phenomenon." *Journal of Homosexuality*, Vol. 34, No. 1 (1997) 73–80.

Byne, William. "Biology and Homosexuality: Implications of neuroendocrinological and neuroanatomical studies." In Robert P. Cabaj and Terry S. Stein, eds. *Textbook of Homo-*

sexuality and Mental Health. Wash., D.C.: American Psychiatric Press (1996) 129–146.

Casey, M. Beth and Ronald L. Nuttall. "Differences in feminine and masculine characteristics in women as a function of handedness: Support for the Geschwind/Galaburda theory of brain organization." *Neuropsychologia,* Vol. 28, No. 7 (1990) 749–754.

Ehret, G. A. and Jurgens et al. "Oestrogen receptor occurrence in the male mouse brain — modulation by paternal experience." *Neuroreport,* Vol. 4, No. 11 (1993) 1247–1250.

Fausto-Sterling, Anne. *Sexing the Body.* New York: Basic Books (Perseus), 2000.

Francis, Darlene and Thomas Insel et al. "Epigenic sources of behavioral differences in mice." *Nature Neuroscience,* Vol. 6, No. 5 (May 2003) 445–446.

Gooren, Louis. "Biomedical theories of sexual orientation: A critical examination." In David P. McWhirter, Stephanie A. Sanders and June M. Reinisch, eds. *Homosexuality/Heterosexuality.* New York: Oxford University Press (1990) 71–77.

Hardy, Marjorie. "The development of gender roles: societal influences." In Louis Diamont and Richard D. McAnulty, eds. *The Psychology of Sexual Orientation, Behavior, and Identity.* Westport, Conn.: Greenwood Press (1995) 424–439.

Harris, Judith Rich. *The Nurture Assumption.* New York: Touchstone (Simon & Shuster) 1999.

Kauth, Michael and Seth C. Kalichman. "Sexual orientation and development: an interactive approach." In Louis Diamont and Richard D. McAnulty, eds. *The Psychology of Sexual Orientation, Behavior and Identity.* Westport, Conn.: Greenwood Press (1995) 81–99.

Lewontin, R.C. *Biology as Ideology.* Concord, Ont.: Anansi Press, 1991.

Lewontin, R.C., Steven Rose and Leon J. Kamin. *Not in Our Genes.* New York: Pantheon (Random House), 1984.

Money, John. *Gay, Straight and In-Between.* Oxford University Press, 1988.

Reinisch, June Machover and Stephanie A. Sanders. "Prenatal hormonal contributions to sex differences in human cognitive and personality development." In A. A. Gerall, ed. *Handbook of Behavioral Neurobiology,* Vol. 11 (1992) 221–243.

Rogers, Leslie. *Sexing the Brain.* London: Weidenfeld & Nicolson, 1999.

Rose, Hilary and Steven, eds. *Alas Poor Darwin: Arguments Against Evolutionary Psychology.* London: Jonathan Cape, 2000.

Segal, Nancy. *Entwined Lives.* London: Penguin, 1999.

Siegel, Daniel J. *The Developing Mind.* New York: The Guilford Press, 1999.

Singh, J. A. L. *Wolf-Children and Feral Man.* New York: Harper, 1942.

Udry, J. R. "Biological limits of gender construction." *American Sociological Review,* Vol. 65 (2000) 443–457.

Ward, Ingeborg L. "Sexual behavior: The product of perinatal hormonal and prepubertal social factors." In Arnold A. Gerall, Howard Moltz and Ingeborg L. Ward, eds. *Sexual Differentiation*, Vol. 11 of *Handbook of Behavioral Neurology*. New York: Plenum Press (1992) 157–180.

Wellings, Kaye. *Sexual Behaviour in Britain: The National Survey of Sexual Attitudes and Lifestyles*. London: Penguin Books, 1994.

CHAPTER 8

Adams, Henry E., Lester Wright and Bethany A. Lohr. "Is homophobia associated with homosexual arousal?" *Journal of Abnormal Psychology*, Vol. 105, No. 31 (1996) 440–445.

Altemeyer, Bob. "Changes in attitudes towards homosexuals." *Journal of Homosexuality*, Vol. 4, No. 2 (2001) 63–75.

Bem, Daryl J. "Exotic becomes erotic: A developmental theory of sexual orientation." *Psychological Review*, Vol. 103, No. 2 (1996) 320–335.

Brooks, David. "We should insist on gay marriage." *New York Times* (Nov. 22, 2003) A15.

Brooks, Geraldine. *Nine Parts of Desire: The Hidden World of Islamic Women*. New York: Anchor Books (Random House), 1996.

Dwyer, Victor. "Not so queer as folk," *Maclean's* (June 23, 2003) 42–44.

Ferguson, Sue. "Tale of a Witch Hunt." *Maclean's* (June 25, 2001) 34–36.

Fone, Byne. *Homophobia: A History*. New York: Metropolitan Books, 2000.

Griffith, Kristin and Michelle Hebl. "The disclosure dilemma for gay men and lesbians: Coming out at work." *Journal of Applied Psychology*, Vol. 14, No. 6 (2002) 1191–1199.

Haldeman, Douglas C. "Sexual orientation conversion therapy for gay men and lesbians: a scientific examination." In John C. Gonsiorak and James D. Weinrich, eds. *Homosexuality: Research Implications for Public Policy*. Newberry Park, Calif.: Sage Publications (1991) 149–160.

Herek, Gregory M. "Homosexuality is NOT a disease." AGLA France Forums, Posts 23, Joined Feb. 24, 2002.

Herek, Gregory M. "Psychological heterosexism in the United States." In Anthony R. D'Augelli and Charlotte Patterson, eds. *Lesbian, Gay and Bisexual Identities Over the Lifespan: Psychological Perspectives*. New York: Oxford University Press (1995) 323.

Herek, Gregory M. "Stigma, prejudice and violence against lesbians and gay men." In John C. Gonsiorak and James D. Weinrich, eds. *Homosexuality: Research Implications for Public Policy*. Newberry Park, Calif.: Sage Publications, 1991.

Herrell, Richard et al. "Sexual orientation and suicidality." *Archives of General Psychiatry*, Vol. 5 (Oct 1999) 867–874.

Hershberger, Scott L. and Anthony R. D'Augelli. "The impact of victimization on the mental health and suicidality of lesbian, gay and bisexual youths." *Developmental Psychology*, Vol. 31, No. 1 (1995) 65–74.

Johnson, Pat. "Catholic hypocrisy on sexual matters plain," *Vancouver Courier*, Aug. 6, 2003.

Lane, Charles. "Landmark case for gay-rights advocates," *Washington Post*, reprinted in the *Vancouver Sun*, March 24, 2003.

Lane, Charles. "Gay bishop wins confirmation," *Washington Post*, reprinted in the *Vancouver Sun*, August 6, 2003.

McCreary Centre Society. "Being out: Lesbian, gay, bisexual and transgender youth in B.C.: An adolescent health survey." 1999.

Rennie, David. "Top U.S. court strikes down ban on sodomy," *Vancouver Sun*, June 27, 2003.

Roughgarden, Joan. *Evolution's Rainbow*. Berkeley: University of California Press, 2004.

Rud, Jeff. "School board backs gay rights," *Times Colonist*, June 24, 2003.

Savin-Williams, Ritch C. "An exploratory study of pubertal maturation timing and self-esteem among gay and bisexual male youth." *Developmental Psychology*, Vol. 31, No. 1 (1995) 56.

Savin-Williams, Ritch. *The New Gay Teenager*. Harvard University Press, 2005.

Spitzer, Robert L. "Can some gay men and lesbians change their sexual orientation?" *Archives of Sexual Behavior*, Vol. 32, No.5 (2003) 403–417.

Sullivan, Andrew. "The Vatican's New Stereotype." *TIME* (Dec. 12, 2005) 56.

The Economist Saturday Review, "The unbearable normalcy of being queer," Jan. 27, 1996.

Tibbetts, Janice. "Corrections must pay for sex change," *The Vancouver Sun*, Feb. 7, 2003.

Vallis, Mary. "Bush to block gay marriage," *Vancouver Sun*, July 31, 2003.

Valpy, Michael. "Why same-sex marriage became a sin." *Globe & Mail*, Aug. 9, 2003.

Van der Meide, Wayne. "Legislating Equality." Washington, D.C.: The Policy Institute of the National Gay and Lesbian Task Force, 2001.

Woolley, Paul. "Moral judgement or homophobia?" *British Journal of Sexual Medicine*, Vol. 25, No. 6 (1998) 4.

Permissions

CHAPTER 1

Excerpt from *Escape from Freedom*, by Erich Fromm. Copyright 1941, 1969 by Erich Fromm. Reprinted by arrangement with Henry Holt and Company.

The Sexual Orientation Quiz is adapted from the Klein Sexual Orientation Grid, with the kind permission of the author, Fritz Klein, M. D., San Diego, Calif.

The Brainsex Test is from BRAINSEX: *The Real Difference Between Men and Women* by Anne Moir and David Jessel (Michael Joseph, 1989. Copyright Anne Moir and David Jessel, 1989. Reprinted with permission from The Penguin Group (UK).

Quotations from *The Invention of Heterosexuality*, 1995, by Jonathan Ned Katz, are reprinted by permission from Penguin Putnam Inc., New York, NY.

CHAPTER 2

The epigraph is from *The Napoleon of Notting Hill*, 1904, by G. K. Chesterton. Reprinted by permission from A. P. Watt Ltd., London, UK, on behalf of the Royal Literary Fund.

Information from The Society for Women's Health Research is reprinted with permission from Sarah Gevers, SWHR, Washington, DC.

CHAPTER 3

The quotations from Ann Landers' column are reprinted with permission from Ann Landers and Creators Syndicate.

The quotation from *The Evolution of Human Sexuality*, 1979, by Donald Symons, is reprinted with permission from Oxford University Press, Inc., New York, N.Y.

The interviews with lesbian and gay parents are printed with the generous permission of Alison Brewin and Vanessa Jacobsen, and of Stanley Alexander and Byron Chiefmoon.

The reference to swingers was from *The Lifestyle* by Terry Gould. Copyright © 1999 by Terry Gould. Reprinted by permission of Random House Canada.

CHAPTER 4

The author and publisher have made every reasonable effort to contact the copyright holders of the epigraph on page 66, but have been unable to do so. The publisher requests that the copyright holders contact them so that the permission requirements can be fulfilled.

The "John" case is reproduced by kind permission of the *British Journal of Sexual Medicine* and of the author, Dr. Lynne Webster, Consultant Psychiatrist, Manchester Royal Infirmary.

The interviews with "Isabella," David Harrison and Danielle Anderson are printed with their kind permission.

CHAPTER 6

The epigraph is from *The Ascent of Man* by Jacob Brownowski, published by Little, Brown and Company in 1974.

CHAPTER 7

The epigraph is from *Texts and Pretexts* by Aldous Huxley, originally published by Chatto and Windus in 1932 © the Estate of Mrs. Laura Huxley. Reprinted here by permission of The Random House Group Limited.

The quotation by Michael Kauth and Seth Kalichman is from *The Psychology of Sexual Orientation, Behaviour and Identity*, Louis Diamont and Richard D. McAnulty, eds., 1995. Reproduced with permission of Greenwood Publishing Group, Inc., Westport, CT.

The quotation from *Advocate*, July 17, 2001, is reprinted with permission from L.A. Liberation Publications, Inc., Los Angeles.

Quotations from Drs. Stephanie Sanders and June Reinisch in the *Handbook of Behavioral Neurology (11)*, 1992, ed. A.A. Gerall, are reprinted by permission of the authors and Kluwer Academic/ Plenum Publisher.

Quotations from Dr. Daniel Siegel in *The Developing Mind*, 1999, are reprinted with permission of The Guilford Press, New York.

CHAPTER 8

The epigraph is from *The True Believer: Thoughts on the Nature of Mass Movements*, 1951, by Eric Hoffer, reprinted by permission of HarperCollins Publishers.

The quotations from Douglas C. Haldeman in *Homosexuality: Research Implications for Public Policy*, 1991, eds. John C. Gonsiorak and James D. Weinrich, are reprinted by permission of the publisher, Sage Publications, Inc.

The "Dear Dr. Laura" letter is reprinted with kind permission of the author, Kent Ashcraft, Bowie, MD, USA.

Information from Alan Yang's report and the 2000 National Elections Study is reprinted with permission from the National Gay and Lesbian Task Force, New York.

The quotation from Dr. Paul Woolley is reproduced by kind permission of the *British Journal of Sexual Medicine*.

Index

adolescent sexuality, 88, 114, 191–92;
    gay, 211, 238
adoption, by same-sex couples, 231, 239,
    242–44
aggression and testosterone, 53–57
aging, brain and, 39–40, 196
ambiguous genitalia, 140–42, 147
American opinion and policies on
    homosexuality, 212–13, 228–36
anal sex, 68, 87
Anderson, Danielle/Danny, 143–46
androgen insensitivity syndrome (AIS),
    17–18
androgen insufficiency, 184, 200; prena-
    tal exposure to, 166, 169–70
animals, homosexuality in, 25–27

Bagemihl, Bruce, 25–27
behaviour, sex differences in, 52–57
Bell, Alan, 84–86
"berdache," 80–81
Bible, homosexuality in the, 221–26
biological basis for sexual orientation,
    105, 172–88. *See also* genetic factors
biological sex differences, 59–61
birth-order, sexual orientation and,
    177–79
birth weight, gay male, 182
bisexuality, 113–22
brain: aging of, 39–40, 196; development
    and prenatal stress, 185–86; division,
    43–50, 160–61, 169, 201; environmen-
    tal influence on, 194; sex differences

in, 36–41, 43–51, 154–59, 161, 169–71;
sex of, 16, 20–21, 22–24
brothers, and sexual orientation, 177–79
"butch" lesbians, 110–11, 167

CAH. *See* congenital adrenal hyperplasia
Canadian opinion and policies on
homosexuality, 213–14, 236–42
Chase, Cheryl, 150, 151–52
childhood, sexual orientation and,
102–3, 123–24, 191–92, 205–8
civil liberties for homosexuals, 228–29,
231–39, 242–45
cognitive abilities, sex differences in,
38–50, 162–64
"coming out," 106, 115, 245–47
communication, sex differences in, 51–52
conception, 35
congenital adrenal hyperplasia (CAH),
16–17
conversion therapy, 218–21
creativity, homosexuality and, 104, 159
criminalization of homosexuality, 211–13,
227–29, 237
cross-dressing, 75–76

DES (diethylstilbestrol), fetal exposure
to, 18–19
developmental instability, 186–87
discrimination: against homosexuals,
212–14, against transsexuals, 139–40.
See also prejudice
DNA, 34
drag kings, 111
drag queens, 91–92
drug reactions, sex differences in, 60
drugs, fetal exposure to, 19
Durand, Sylvie/Sylvain, 134–35

effeminacy, 102–4
environmental factors in sexual orientation, 193–209
estrogen, 40–50, 56–57, 131–32
exhibitionism, 77–78
experimentation, sexual, 114, 191–92

family influence, 9, 128–29, 202–4
female brain, 20, 21, 38
femininity, measuring, 89
"femme" lesbians, 110–11, 167
fetal development, 194–95; drugs and,
18–19; hormones and, 14–19, 45,
50–51, 115–19, 165–70, 183–84; 197,
199; maternal antibodies and, 181–83;
sexual orientation and, 115, 119,
165–66, 181–85, 187, 191; ultrasound
and, 186–87
"fetal wastage" theory, 182–83
fetishism, sexual, 77
finger length, differences in, 58, 167
fingertip ridges, differences in, 57–58,
166–67
5-alpha Reductase Deficiency, 19
"flashers," 77–78
Freund, Kurt, 66

gay-bashing. *See* violence against
homosexuals
gay marriage. *See* same-sex marriage
gay parenting, 95–102
gay/straight differences, 154–59, 161,
162–67
"gender-bending," 123
gender clinics, 131, 133
gender, definition of, 3–4, 30
gender dysphoria, 122–40. *See also*
transsexuals

Gender Identity Disorder (GID), 124
gender nonconformity, childhood, 102–3
genetic evolution, 34–35
genetic factors in sexual orientation,
    157–58, 174–81, 182–83, 193–209
genital ambiguity, 140–42, 147
genital size, 168–69
Gould, Terry, 71–72

Haldeman, Douglas, 219–20
hand preference, 105, 159–61, 169, 186–87
hate-crime laws, homosexuality and, 228, 238
hearing, sex differences in, 41, 165–66
hermaphrodites. See intersexuals
heterosexual sexuality, 65–70, 79–80,
    114, 191–92
homophobia, 210–47; and suppressed
    homosexual desire, 214–15
homosexual, definition of, 79
homosexuality: in animals, 25–27;
    and creativity, 104, 159; criminal-
    ization of, 211–13, 227–29, 237;
    factors in, 157–58, 187, 190–92, 198;
    family influence on, 92–95, 102–3;
    incidence of, 80–83, 86, 103–4;
    medicalization of, 215–16, 218–21;
    myths about, 215–18; religious
    objections to, 221–27; violence
    against, 211–14
hormones: cognitive abilities and, 45,
    48–49, 50–51, 55, 105; effect on
    behaviour of, 55–56; fetal exposure
    to, 14–15, 165–66, 168–69, 183–84;
    insufficiency, 184, 200; stress, 60–61,
    184–85; syndromes caused by, 16–19;
    therapy for gender dysphoria,
    131–32

hypothalamus, sex difference in the,
    20–21, 41
identical twins, 167–68, 174–76
immune response, homosexuality and
    maternal, 181–83
immune system, sex differences in, 42
incidence: of bisexuality, 119–20;
    homosexuality, 81–83, 86, 103–4;
    intersexuality, 141; transsexuality,
    129
infancy, sex differences in, 53
intersexuals, 140–52

Johnston, Jack, 137–38
Jorgensen, Christine, 130

Kinsey, Alfred, 82–83
Kinsey reports, 82–83

language skills, 46; sex differences in,
    38, 47, 49, 50, 162
law, homosexuality and the, 211–14,
    227–32, 236–40, 242–45
left-handedness, 105, 159–61, 169,
    186–87
lesbian parenting, 95–99, 231
lesbianism, 81, 82, 106–7, 108–10;
    biological basis for, 56, 105, 154,
    165–67, 179; social basis for, 107–8
libido, 24–25, 70, 90–91, 109

marriage, same-sex, 221, 228–31, 239–44
masculinity, measuring, 89, 168
masturbation, frequency of, 67–68, 87
men, hormone levels in, 55, 56–57
mental health: and "coming out,"
    245–46; of gay and lesbian teens,
    211; of homosexuals, 84–86;

of intersexuals, 142–43; of transsexuals, 128, 136, 139–40
mental illness, treatment of homosexuality as, 215–16, 218–21
mental skills, sex differences in, 38–50, 162–64
Money, John, 147
myths about homosexuality, 215–18

navigation, sex differences in, 47–49
neurosteroids, 184

oral sex, frequency of, 68–69, 87, 108
orgasm, rates of, 69

paraphiliacs, 76–78
parental influence. *See* family influence
parenting, same-sex, 95–102
pedophilia, 78–79, 217
physical sex differences, 41–42, 57–61, 164–68
physiological sex differences, 59–61
plethysmograph, 66
political basis for sexual orientation, 107–8, 120, 121
prejudice: against homosexuals, 211–14, 215–17; 221–36; against transsexuals, 139–40
prenatal development, 194–95; drugs and, 18–19; hormones and, 14–19, 45, 50–51, 115–19, 165–70, 183–84, 197, 199; maternal antibodies and, 181–83; sexual orientation and, 115, 119, 165–66, 181–85, 187, 191; ultrasound and, 186–87
prostitution, gay youth in, 211
puberty, onset of, 165
rates of: bisexuality, 119–20;

homosexuality, 81–83, 86, 103–4; intersexuality, 141; transsexuality, 129
Reimer, Bruce/Brenda (David), 147, 149–50
religious objections to homosexuality, 221–27
right-handedness and fetal development, 186

same-sex marriage, 221, 228–31, 239–44
same-sex parenting, 95–102
same-sex sexual experience, 79 80, 88, 114, 191–92
sex-change surgery, 130, 132–36
sex, definition of, 30
sex differences: in behaviour, 52–57; in brain, 20–21, 36–41, 47–51; in infancy, 53; in libido, 70, 90–91, 109; physical, 41–42, 57–61, 164–68; sensory differences, 41–42, 165–66
sex drive, 24–25, 27, 70, 90–91, 109
sex, frequency of, 87, 109, 119
sexual experimentation, 114, 191–92
sexual identity, 30, 147–50
sexual orientation, 30, 124; biological basis for, 172–88; environmental factors in, 205–8; quiz, 28–29; social construction of, 190–92
sexual partners, number of, 67, 90–91
sexual preferences, unusual, 76–77
sleep patterns, homosexual, 155
smell, sex differences in sense of, 41
Smith, Frances/Arnell, 138
sodomy laws, 212–13
spatial skills, 47–51, 162
spousal benefits for homosexual couples, 232, 237, 239

startle response, gay/straight differences in, 166
stereotypes of homosexuals, 216–17
stress hormones, 60–61, 184–85
Stuart, Jenna, 137–38
suicide rates in homosexual teens, 211
Sullivan, Andrew, 54
surgery, sex-change, 130, 132–36, 239
surgical alteration of infant intersexuals, 141–43, 147, 150–51, 152
"swinging," 70–74

testosterone, 53–57, 132, 183; prenatal exposure to, 45, 50–51, 169, 199
"transgender," 4, 122
transsexuals, 122–40, 169–71, 239
transvestism, 75–76

twins, 165–66, 167–68, 174–76

U.S. opinion and policies on homosexuality, 212–13, 228–36
ultrasound, fetal exposure to, 186–87

violence against homosexuals, 211–14
voyeurism, 77

Weinberg, Martin, 84–86
"wife-swapping," 70–74
Witelson, Sandra, 158–59
women, testosterone levels in, 56

x chromosome, 59

y chromosome, 59

About the Author

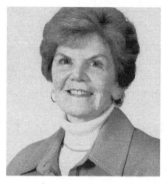

OLIVE SKENE JOHNSON is a retired neuro-psychologist, clinician and author who for many years operated a private Psychology practice in Vancouver. She received a B.A. degree in English and History from the University of British Columbia, a B.A.(Hons.) degree and a Master of Science degree (both in Psychology) from Memorial University of Newfoundland, and a Ph.D. degree in Psychology from the University of British Columbia. She is a past member of The National Academy of Neuropsychology (U.S.) In addition to academic publications, her articles have appeared in popular magazines including *McCall's, Macleans, Chatelaine, Vancouver Life and Queens.* The mother of three sons and two daughters, Dr. Johnson lives with her husband, Ross, in Vancouver.

By printing **The Sexual Spectrum** on paper made from 100% post-consumer recycled fibre rather than virgin tree fibre, Raincoast Books has made the following ecological savings:

- 22 trees
- 872 kilograms of greenhouse gases (equivalent to driving an average North American car for two months)
- 15 million BTUs (equivalent to the power consumption of a North American home for two months)
- 30,226 litres of water (equivalent to nearly one Olympic sized pool)
- 464 kilograms of solid waste (equivalent to nearly one garbage truck load)

(Environmental impact estimates were made using the Environmental Defense Paper Calculator. For more information, visit http://www.papercalculator.org.)

RAINCOAST BOOKS
www.raincoast.com

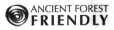